Instructor's Manual to Accompany

Fundamentals of Nursing: The Art and Science of Nursing Care

Second Edition

Carol Taylor, CSFN, RN, MSN, PhD (candidate)
Assistant Professor, Nursing
Georgetown University
Washington, DC
Holy Family College
Philadelphia, PA

Carol Lillis, RN, MSN
Associate Professor
Department of Nursing
Delaware County Community College
Media, PA

Priscilla LeMone, RNC, DSN
Assistant Professor
University of Missouri - Columbia
Columbia, MO

J.B. Lippincott Company
Philadelphia

Sponsoring Editor: Donna L. Hilton, RN, BSN
Coordinating Editorial Assistant: Susan Perry
Production Coordinator: Nannette Winski
Production Manager: Helen Ewan

Desktop Composition: Harp Associates
Printer/Binder: Capital City Press
Cover Printer: Lehigh Press

1 3 5 6 4 2

ISBN 0-397-54949-0

Any procedure or practice described in this book should be applied by the health-care practitioner under appropriate supervision in accordance with professional standards of care used with regard to the unique circumstances that apply in each practice situation. Care has been taken to confirm the accuracy of information presented and to describe generally accepted practices. However, the authors, editors, and publisher cannot accept any responsibility for errors or omissions or for any consequences from application of the information in this book and make no warranty, express or implied, with respect to the contents of the book.

Every effort has been made to ensure drug selections and dosages are in accordance with current recommendations and practice. Because of ongoing research, changes in government regulations and the constant flow of information on drug therapy, reactions and interactions, the reader is cautioned to check the package insert for each drug for indications, dosages, warnings and precautions, particularly if the drug is new or infrequently used.

Instructor's Manual to Accompany

Fundamentals of Nursing:
The Art and Science of Nursing Care

Introduction

This instructor's manual for the second edition of <u>Fundamentals of Nursing: The Art and Science of Nursing Care</u> is designed to provide classroom, learning laboratory, and clinical application resources for instructors of Fundamentals of Nursing courses. The manual provides content and teaching/learning activities for each chapter of the book. Objectives and activities are written to encompass the cognitive, psychomotor, and affective domains, based on the belief of the authors that student learning is increased when a variety of learning experiences are used. This variety of teaching resources will also facilitate adaptation to individualized preferences in teaching methods and learning requirements.

The chapters correlate to those in the text and the following format is used, as applicable, for each chapter:

Learner Objectives

These chapter objectives, included at the beginning of each chapter, focus content on student learning and describe expected outcomes following mastery of chapter content.

Key Terms

The key terms, listed at the beginning of each chapter, are defined within the textbook chapter and in the Glossary at the end of the text. The key term is boldfaced in the textbook the first time it is defined.

Key Topics

The key topics provide a brief topical summary of the chapter and provide information about the major concepts and skills covered in the chapter.

Recurring Displays

Recurring displays are boxed materials that reappear throughout the book. Although each display is not included in every chapter, the titles remain constant throughout while the information changes specific to the content of the chapter. The recurring displays for this edition of the book are:

- Research in Nursing: Making a Difference
- Focus on the Older Adult
- Nursing Today: Challenges and Solutions
- Focused Assessment Guides
- Computer Applications in Nursing
- Through the Eyes of a Student
- Promoting Wellness
- Guidelines for Nursing Care
- Nursing Diagnoses for Common Problems
- Nursing Process in Clinical Practice

Other Significant Displays and Tables

The section of other significant displays and tables includes tables, boxed material, and forms used within the chapter to supplement information found in the narrative text. This list is provided to highlight important content useful to the instructor.

Procedures

Procedures included in the textbook chapter are listed so that the instructor has a quick reference when making assignments and lesson plans.

Nursing Process in Clinical Practice

Each chapter in Unit IV of the text concludes with a case study and care plan specific for the person described in the clinical scenario. A brief description of the individual and the nursing diagnoses are provided here.

Teaching-Learning Activities

The teaching-learning activities are divided into three areas:

Group Activities: These activities include

- exercises, discussion topics, presentations,
- experiences, learning laboratory practice, and
- clinical application. They facilitate student
- learning through application of chapter content
- in structured or guided observational experiences.

Discussion Questions: The discussion questions provide recall, application, and analysis of chapter content through verbal discussion. Discussion questions also facilitate practice with critical-thinking and problem-solving abilities.

Writing Activities: The writing activities include a variety of activities designed to assist students in integrating chapter content while improving written expression skills. The emphasis on writing abilities in higher education requires that writing activities be an integral component across the curriculum.

Contents

Chapter 1
Introduction to Nursing

Learner Objectives

- Define key terms used in the chapter.
- Describe the historical background, the definitions of nursing, and the status of nursing as a profession and as a discipline.
- Identify the aims of nursing as they interrelate to facilitate maximum function and quality of life for clients.
- Describe the various levels of educational preparation in nursing.
- Discuss the effect of nursing organizations, standards of nursing practice, nurse practice acts, and the nursing process on the practice of nursing.
- Identify current trends in nursing.

Key Terms

Continuing education
Dependent nursing actions
Discipline
Holistic health care
Independent nursing actions
In-service education
Interdependent nursing actions
Licensure

Nurse Practice Act
Nursing
Nursing Education
Nursing process
Profession
Standard
Wellness

Key Topics

Nursing: An emerging profession: historical background, nursing in North America, definitions, a profession or a discipline, aims.

Educational preparation for nursing practice: levels of education, continuing education, in-service education.

Professional nursing organizations: national, international, specialty.

Guidelines for nursing practice: standards, nurse practice acts and licensure, nursing process.

Nursing in transition: new directions, changes in client needs, increased responsibility.

Significant Displays and Tables

Competencies of the Associate Degree Nurse on Entry into Practice
Competencies of the Graduate of the Baccalaureate Program in Nursing
American Nurses' Association Standards of Clinical Nursing Practice
Canadian Nurses' Association Standards of Nursing Practice

Teaching-Learning Activities

Group Activities

1. Divide the class into groups of two or three students and have each group select an educational level and a decade; then each group will interview a nurse meeting those criteria and report back to the class.

2. Ask nurses who are active members of nursing organizations to give a panel presentation about membership and functions. Include a member of the student nurse association.

3. Give each student a copy of the nurse practice act of your state or province and discuss the contents of the law.

4. Discuss the social policy statement of the American Nurses' Association (1980). Choose students to represent the "pros" and another the "cons" for the policy and have a debate.

Discussion Questions

1. How has the historical background of nursing influenced the structure, responsibilities, and aims of nursing today?

2. Should nurses who do not meet established standards of practice work in the clinical setting? If not, what control is available?

3. Is nursing a discipline or a profession (or both). Explain your answer.

4. How does an increasingly elderly population affect a person's future career as a nurse?

Writing Activities

1. Ask students to write a paragraph defining nursing from personal perspectives and experiences.

2. Ask students to choose one of the broad aims of nursing and describe activities they have seen nurses do to meet that aim.

3. Compare and contrast the three types of nursing actions: dependent, interdependent, independent. Do these labels have the same meaning as others in use, such as nurse-initiated actions and physician-initiated orders?

Chapter 2
Promoting Wellness in Health and Illness

Learner Objectives

- Define key terms used in the chapter.
- Describe wellness, health, and illness.
- Identify the factors influencing health and illness, including the human dimensions, basic human needs, and self-concept.
- Compare and contrast acute illness and chronic illness.
- Summarize the role of the nurse in promoting wellness based on knowledge of risk factors for illness, illness behaviors, and the effects of illness on the family.
- Describe the levels of preventive care.

Key Terms

Acute Illness
Agent-host-environment model
Basic human needs
Chronic illness
Disease
Health
Health-belief model

Health-illness continuum
High-level wellness
Illness
Primary preventive care
Risk factor
Secondary preventive care
Tertiary preventive care

Key Topics

Defining wellness in health and illness.

Models of health and illness: the health-illness continuum, high-level wellness model, agent-host-environment model, health-belief model.

Factors affecting health and illness: Factors influencing health-illness status, beliefs, and practices (physical, emotional, intellectual, environmental, sociocultural, and spiritual dimensions); basic human needs; self-concept.

Promoting wellness and preventing illness: risk factors, acute and chronic illness, effects of illness on the family.

Nursing care as preventive care: levels of preventive care (primary, secondary, tertiary), nurse as role model.

Recurring Displays

Nursing Today: Health Promotion.
Focus on the Older Adult: Risk Factors for Illness and Injury in the Older Adult.

Other Significant Displays and Tables

Major Areas of Risk Factors (Table 2.1)
Healthstyle: A Self-test

Teaching-Learning Activities

Group Activities

1. Divide the class into four groups. Ask each group to use one of the health models to illustrate application for different age groups and illnesses. Provide students with examples, such as a 15-year-old with a fractured arm, a 55-year-old with an ulcer, and a 75-year-old with heart problems. Each group will share with the class.

2. Have students meet in small groups to discuss how experiences as members of a family affected the students' own health status, beliefs, and practices.

3. Ask each student to individually complete a health appraisal and share the results in small group discussion.

4. Ask the wellness program director at a local agency to discuss the program with the class.

Discussion Questions

1. What are the implications of "holistic" health care for nursing in today's society?

2. How can lifestyle affect wellness? Consider diet, exercise, rest and sleep, stress, chemical dependency.

3. Compare the environment of a resident of a large city with that of a rural resident. What risk factors are present in each setting?

4. How can the nurse serve as a role model for health? Ask students to identify their own behaviors that will help clients develop or maintain healthy behaviors.

Writing Activities

1. Ask students to write a paragraph that describes their personal definition of health.

2. Compare and contrast these terms: health, wellness, illness, disease.

3. Ask students to describe their own illness behaviors and how these behaviors were influenced by family values and beliefs as well by own personal values and priorities.

4. Ask students to make a list of preventive care activities available in the community that are advertised in the phone book, local newspaper(s), radio, and television.

Chapter 3
The Health Care System

Learner Objectives

- Define key terms used in the chapter.
- Compare and contrast in-patient and out-patient health care settings.
- Discuss the services provided by community health care agencies and in community settings.
- Describe government health care agencies and services.
- Describe the roles of members of the health care team.
- Discuss various private insurance, group plans, and federal support in the United States and Canada.
- Discuss trends and issues affecting the health care delivery system.

Key Terms

Crisis intervention centers

Day-care centers

Diagnosis-related groups

Health maintenance organization

Hospice

Inpatient

Medicaid

Medicare

Preferred provider arrangement

Preferred provider organization

Public Health Service

Key Topics

Types of health care settings: inpatient, extended care facilities, out-patient, physician's offices, clinics and ambulatory centers, community centers, home care agencies, day-care centers, crisis intervention centers, community agencies, hospices, government agencies, voluntary agencies, home care.

The health care team.

The economics of health care delivery: private insurance, group plans, long-term care insurance.

Federal government health care support: United States (Medicare, diagnosis-related groups), Canada.

Trends and issues in the health care delivery system: focus on self-care and wellness, consumer movement, cost-containment, fragmentation of care, increasing numbers of older and chronically ill adults, health care: a right or a privilege?

Recurring Displays

Computer Applications: Computer Use in Hospitals to Reduce Health Care Costs.
Nursing Today: Nursing in the Community.

Teaching-Learning Activities

Group Activities

1. Ask the administrator of a local health care agency or institution to discuss the economics of the setting.

2. Have representatives of different health care settings give a panel presentation that describes the role of the nurse in each setting.

3. Have the class divide in half and debate the advantages and disadvantages of DRGs.

Discussion Questions

1. How do health maintenance organizations promote wellness?

2. What is the future for growth of health care settings for the elderly, such as adult day-care centers, extended care facilities, and respite care?

3. What happens to the person who has no insurance and is injured or becomes ill? Who should pay for this care? Is health care a right or a privilege?

4. What is meant by the phrase "fragmentation of care"? How does the phenomenon affect the client, especially the client who is older and chronically ill?

Writing Activities

1. Ask students to list the different types of health care settings they have experienced or observed and briefly describe their differences and similarities.

2. Ask students to summarize the major points of an article that discusses DRGs.

3. Ask students to choose one type of practice setting and give examples of the nurse's role and functions in that setting.

Chapter 4
Theoretical Base for Nursing Practice

Learner Objectives

- Define key terms used in the chapter.
- Describe the underlying processes and characteristics of nursing theory.
- Define the four common components of nursing theory.
- Summarize the historical background, cultural influences, and value of nursing theory.
- Discuss selected nursing theories, including definitions, assumptions, beliefs, and applications to nursing practice.

Key Terms

Adaptation theory	Nursing theory
Concept	Philosophy
Conceptual framework or model	Process
Developmental theory	Theory
General systems theory	

Key Topics

An introduction to theory.

Nursing theory: basic processes in the development of nursing theories, general systems theory, stress/adaptation theory, basic characteristics of nursing theory, common components.

Nursing theory and nursing practice: historical perspectives and influences, nursing in the United States, developing a scientific base for nursing.

Evolution of nursing theory: research and publishing, educational advances in nursing.

Value of nursing theory: broad goals, application to practice, communication, autonomy.

Conceptual and theoretical frameworks for nursing:

Theorists and their models: (Johnson, King, Leininger, Levine, B. Newman, Orem, Rogers, Roy, Watson), application.

Significant Displays and Tables

Case Study: Julie Smith - Applying Conceptual and Theoretical Frameworks
Theorists and Their Conceptual Models (Table 4.1)

Teaching-Learning Activities

Group Activities

1. Divide the class into small groups and assign each group one or two of the nursing theorists discussed in the chapter. Ask each group to compose one paragraph describing the beliefs about nursing of the assigned theorist(s).

2. Ask students to work together in groups to summarize the theoretical model or conceptual framework of a theorist not included in the chapter.

Discussion Questions

1. What is the difference between a theory and a conceptual framework?

2. How have changes in women's rights influenced theory development in nursing?

3. Defend the following statement "Nursing theory improves and facilitates communication in nursing."

Writing Activities

1. Ask students to write their own definitions of the four concepts common to nursing theory: person, environment, health, nursing.

2. Ask students to choose one nursing theorist and describe how that person's theory or concepts can be applied to themselves when they are well and when they are ill.

Chapter 5
Values and Ethics in Nursing

Learner Objectives

- Define key terms used in the chapter.
- List five common modes of value transmission.
- Identify the seven basic values essential in the practice of nursing.
- Describe seven steps in the valuing process.
- Utilize values clarification strategies in clinical practice.
- Identify three sources of standards for professional ethical conduct.
- Describe nursing practice which is consistent with the code of ethics for nursing.
- Describe three typical concerns of the nurse advocate.
- Recognize ethical issues as they arise in nursing practice.
- Utilize an ethical framework and decision making process to resolve ethical problems.
- Identify four functions of institutional ethics committees.

Key Terms

Advocacy	Fidelity
Attitude	Justice
Autonomy	Morals
Beliefs	Nursing ethics
Beneficence	Nonmaleficence
Biomedical ethics	Paternalism
Confidentiality	Utilitarianism
Decontological	Value
Ethics	Value system
Ethics committee	Values clarification
Ethics of caring	Veracity

Key Topics

Values: types of values, development of values, values essential to the professional nurse, values clarification.

Ethics: professional ethical conduct, advocacy, types of moral and ethical problems, ethical decision making, nurses and ethics committees.

Recurring Displays

Computer Applications in Nursing: Computer Program, "Dr. Ethics," which analyzes the ethical implications of case studies in clinical medicine

Through the Eyes of a Student

Other Significant Displays and Tables

Essential values, attitudes and personal qualities of the professional nurse (Table 5-1)

Example of the valuing process

Three Codes of Ethics for Nurses (ICN, ANA, CNA)

A Patient's Bill of Rights

A Case Study Using a Six Step Process for Resolving Ethical Problems

Thirteen mini-cases are presented in this chapter (under the heading "Types of Moral and Ethical Problems) which illustrate typical ethical problems nurses encounter in their professional practice. Students are invited to role-play these situations and evaluate the courses of action they take.

Teaching-Learning Activities

Group Activities

1. Divide the class in half and have them debate the values and ethics of a current issue, such as maintaining life to preserve organs for transplant.

2. Ask students individually to write down the five most important parts of their lives and then share them in small groups. Encourage exploration of priorities and choices.

3. Ask students to determine their course of action as the nurse in the situation listed below. Consider the patient's rights. Divide the class into small groups to share their thoughts.

   Mr. Monroe is an eighty-year-old man admitted to your unit from a nursing home. He requires treatment for complications of his diabetes. Mr. Monroe is visually impaired and he has had a below-the-knee amputation of his right leg. Several toes are gangrenous and require amputation. Mr. Monroe is refusing to consent to this surgery. He has stated: "Go away and let me die."

4. Have the class as a group discuss family and cultural influences on each student's values. Use sample situations in Chapter five.

Discussion Questions

1. How would you use the six-step ethical problem-solving process to evaluate your actions when an assigned client says: "I'm afraid I have a venereal disease, but please don't tell anyone"?

2. How would your own values influence your nursing care for clients who are (a) injured while under the influence of drugs or alcohol, (b) have AIDS, (c) are addicted to drugs, (d) have an abortion.

3. Should nurses support the Patient's Bill of Rights? Defend your answer.

4. What does informed consent mean for clients? For nurses?

Writing Activities

1. Have students write a paragraph about nursing using these words: value, value system, attitude, belief.

2. Ask students to write out the conversation they would have, based on values clarification and ethical decision making, if their best friend and fellow student nurse confided: "I can only handle client care if I smoke pot."

3. Have the students select the three values which are most important to them and the three values which are least important to them from the list below and write a paragraph explaining their choices.

respect	responsibility	education
glamour	authority	work
drama	creativity	traditions
autonomy	financial security	health
independence	status	marriage

Chapter 6
Legal Implications of Nursing

Learner Objectives

- Define key terms used in the chapter.
- Define law, describing its four sources.
- Describe the professional and legal regulation of nursingpractice.
- Identify the purpose of credentialing; using as examplesaccreditation, licensure/registration, and certification.
- Differentiate intentional torts (assault and battery, defamation, invasion of privacy, false imprisonment, fraud) and unintentional torts (negligence).
- Evaluate personal areas of potential liability in nursing.
- Describe the legal procedure once a plaintiff files a complaint against a nurse for negligence.
- Describe the roles of the nurse as defendant, fact witness, and expert witness.
- Utilize appropriate legal safeguards in nursing practice.
- Explain the purpose of incident reports.
- Describe laws affecting nursing practice.

Key Terms

Accredidation	Expert Witness	Litigation
Advance directive	Fact Witness for health care	Living will
Assault	False Imprisonment	Malpractice
Battery	Felony	Misdemeanor
Certification	Fraud	Negligence
Civil law	Incident report	Plaintiff
Common law	Informed consent	Public law
Crime	Invasion of privacy	Risk management
Defamation of character	Law	Standard of care
Defendant	Liability	Statutory law
Durable power of attorney	Licensure	Tort

Key Topics

Legal concepts: sources of law, litigation

Professional and legal regulation of nursing practice: credentialing

Crimes and torts: intentional torts, unintentional torts

Legal safeguards for the nurse: contracts, competent practice, executing physician orders, documentation, adequate staffing, professional liability insurance, risk management programs, incident reports, Good Samaritan laws

Student liability

Laws affecting nursing practice: occupational safety and health, reporting obligations, controlled substances, wills

Legal issues related to death and dying: advance directives, do not resuscitate (DNR), no code orders

Significant Displays and Tables

Areas of Potential Liability for Nurses (Table 6-2)

Nursing Malpractice Prevention (Table 6-3)

Sample Living Will (Table 6-5)

Sample Durable Power of Attorney for Health Care (Table 6-6)

Checklist to Ensure Informed Consent

Teaching-Learning Activities

Group Activities

1. Ask a lawyer or hospital risk manager to discuss legal implications of health care and nursing.

2. Review forms and discuss situations where the following might be used: incident forms, informed consent forms, leaving the hospital against medical advice (AMA).

3. Discuss the components of your state's or province's nurse practice act with your instructor.

4. Have students work in small groups to discuss a recent nursing journal article that described specific legal cases; ask groups to consider how these legal difficulties could have been avoided. Invite a nurse defendant or nursing expert to share their experiences.

Discussion Questions:

1. When should a nurse question a physician's order? What is the correct procedure for questioning a physician's order?

2. Does the nurse practice act for your state or province define specific areas that would cause loss of licensure? What are those areas?

3. What is the difference between a crime and tort? Give some examples of each that relate to nursing.

4. How is a licensed professional nurse defined in your state or province and what is the licensed professional nurse permitted to do?

Writing Activities

1. Ask students to outline the responsibilities of the nurse who is to be part of a trial.

2. Have students describe their feelings about no-code and slow-code orders. Ask them to consider this issue from their own viewpoint as nurses, and from the viewpoint of a family member of a terminally-ill client.

3. Ask students to make a list of behaviors and activities that would result in legal action against a nurse in your state or province.

4. Ask students to compare and contrast licensure and certification.

Chapter 7

Basic Human Needs:
Individual, Family, and Community

Learner Objectives

- Define key terms used in the chapter.
- Describe each level of Maslow's hierarchy of basic human needs.
- Discuss nursing actions necessary to meet needs for each level of Maslow's hierarchy.
- Discuss family concepts, including family roles, structures, functions, developmental stages, tasks, and health risk factors.
- Identify aspects of the community that affect individual and family health.
- Describe nursing interventions to promote and maintain wellness in the individual as a member of a family and as a member of the community.

Key Terms

Basic human needs	Physiologic needs
Blended family	Safety and security needs
Cohabiting family	Self-actualization needs
Community	Self-esteem needs
Extended family	Single-parent family
Hierarchy of basic needs	Step-family
Love and belonging needs	Traditional family
Nuclear family	

Key Topics

The individual: levels of needs, applying Maslow's theory.

The family: what is a family?, family structures, family functions, developmental tasks, the family in health and illness (risk factors, nursing interventions to promote wellness).

The community: risk factors, nursing in the community.

Recurring Displays

Research in Nursing: Basic Human Needs
Nursing Diagnoses: The Family

© 1993 J.B. Lippincott Co., Fundamentals of Nursing:
The Art and Science of Nursing Care

Other Significant Displays and Tables

Family Stages and Tasks (Table 7.1)

Nursing Interventions to Promote Wellness (Table 7.2)

Teaching-Learning Activities

Group Activities

1. Divide the class into small groups to discuss basic human needs as they apply to each person in the group at a different time (for example, when studying, ill, or under stress). Include situations when higher order needs took precedence.

2. Ask the class to discuss family roles and structure within the family of each student. Consider how these differ from those of parents and grandparents.

3. Ask a social worker or community health nurse to present community influences that are major risk factors for the health of individuals and families.

Discussion Questions

1. What problems do single-parent families face that are different from those faced by the traditional family?

2. Are the tasks for family survival and continuity as defined by Duvall appropriate in today's society? What should be added or deleted?

3. What nursing actions can be used to promote wellness in the family?

4. What community resources are available to promote wellness in individuals and families?

Writing Activities

1. Ask students to write a short autobiographical description of how they learned the health beliefs and practices necessary to satisfy their basic human needs.

2. Ask individual students to describe their feelings and responses to a situation in which they lost self-esteem.

3. Ask students to list five rules learned in their family that promoted good health (for example, "wash your hands before you eat").

Chapter 8
Culture and Ethnicity

Learner Objectives

- Define key terms used in the chapter.
- Discuss the concepts of culture, ethnicity, race, and stereotyping.
- Describe cultural and ethnic characteristics that influence health care, including gender roles, language and communication, orientation to space and time, food and nutrition, socioeconomic factors, importance of family, physical and mental characteristics, spiritual characteristics, and perceptions of illness and health.
- Compare and contrast the culture of the health care system with the broad concept of culture.
- Identify the factors that affect the interaction of the nurse and the client in terms of health care values.
- Discuss the guidelines that are useful in practicing transcultural nursing care.
- Use knowledge of specific cultural and ethnic factors in providing holistic, individualized nursing care to clients.

Key Terms

Cultural imposition	Minority group
Cultural assimilation	Personal space
Culture	Race
Culture shock	Stereotyping
Dominant group	Subculture
Ethnicity	Transcultural nursing
Ethnocentrism	Yin and Yang

Key Topics

Concepts of culture and ethnicity: culture, cultural assimilation, ethnicity, race, stereotyping.

Cultural and ethnic influences on health care: gender roles, language and communication, orientation to space and time, food and nutrition, socioeconomic factors, family support, physical and mental health, folk medicine.

Transcultural nursing: the culture of health care, cultural imposition and ethnocentrism, providing transcultural care.

Recurring Displays

Research in Nursing: Culture

Through the Eyes of a Student

Nursing Diagnoses: Culture and Ethnicity

Other Significant Displays and Tables

Cultural Factors Affecting Nursing Care (Table 8.1)

Cultural Norms of the Healthcare System

Teaching-Learning Activities

Group Activities

1. Discuss cultural and ethnic differences in the community, using definitions such as old/young, poor/wealthy, and rural/urban, as well as traditional definitions.

2. Ask a faculty member or a student of a cultural or racial minority to speak about both positive and negative aspects of life as a member of a minority group.

3. Assign groups of two or three students to learn basic words and phrases in a language other than their own that are necessary to health care and present them to the class.

Discussion Questions

1. What are some commonly used examples of stereotyping? How are nurses stereotyped? How can this practice affect health care?

2. What are the differences among race, ethnic group, and culture?

3. Discuss the statement "The health care system is a culture". Do you agree or disagree and why?

4. Can feelings on entering nursing school be compared to culture shock? How does "burn-out" in practicing nurses compare to culture shock?

Writing activities

1. Have each student pretend to be elderly and living on a fixed income. Suddenly surgery is required. What feelings would be experienced?

2. Ask students to research literature on one of the illnesses specific to certain ethnic groups and write a more complete description of symptoms and treatment.

3. Ask students to summarize a recent nursing journal article that describes an area of transcultural nursing.

Chapter 9
Stress and Adaptation

Learner Objectives

- Define key terms used in the chapter.
- Describe the mechanisms involved in maintaining physiologic homeostasis.
- Explain the interdependent nature of stressors, stress, and adaptation.
- Compare and contrast developmental and situational stress, incorporating the concepts of physiologic and psychosocial stressors.
- Describe the physical and emotional responses to stress, including mind-body interaction, local adaptation syndrome, general adaptation syndrome, and coping/defense mechanisms.
- Discuss the effects of short- and long-term stress on basic human needs, health and illness, and the family.
- Integrate knowledge of healthy lifestyle, support systems, stress management techniques, and crisis intervention into nursing care plans.
- Recognize and effectively cope with stress unique to the nursing profession.

Key Terms

Adaptation	General adaptation syndrome (GAS)
Anxiety	Homeostasis
Burnout	Inflammatory response
Caregiver burden	Local adaptation syndrome (LAS)
Coping mechanisms	Psychosomatic disorders
Crisis	Reflex pain response
Crisis intervention	Situational stress
Defense mechanisms	Stress
Developmental crisis	Stressor
"Flight or fight" response	

Key Topics

Homeostasis: physiologic, psychologic.

Basic concepts of stress and adaptation: definitions, dimensions of stress and adaptation.

Adaptation: Responses to stress: mind-body interaction, physiologic responses to stress (GAS, LAS), psychosocial responses to stress.

Effects of stress: interaction with basic human needs, stress in health and illness, family reactions, prolonged stress, crisis.

Nursing actions to promote stress reduction: activities of daily living, support systems, stress management techniques, crisis intervention.

Stress management for nurses.

Recurring Displays

Research in Nursing: Stress and Adaptation
Nursing Today: The Homeless
Nursing Diagnoses: Stress and Adaptation

Other Significant Displays and Tables

Social Readjustment Rating Scale (Table 9.2)
Relaxation Activities

Teaching-Learning Activities

Group Activities

1. Ask students to share individual physical and emotional responses to stress and to identify coping mechanism used.
2. Ask students to individually complete the Social Readjustment Rating Scale and then to compare scores in small groups.
3. Ask a mental health nurse to lead students in stress reduction activities.

Discussion Questions

1. How do the reflex pain response and the inflammatory response help maintain homeostasis?
2. Describe the stages of GAS and explain how they were manifested in clients being cared for.
3. What defense mechanisms do you use to cope with stress? Are these healthy or unhealthy?
4. Do you personally know a nurse who has experienced burnout? If so, how did they feel and respond?

Writing Activities

1. Ask students to choose one of the defense mechanisms described in the chapter and write a description of the stressor that precipitated it in themselves, a friend, or a family member.
2. Ask students to list the stressors they have observed to affect hospitalized clients.
3. Ask students to choose a time in their life when they felt they were in a crisis situation and apply the five steps of crisis intervention.

Chapter 10
Developmental Concepts

Learner Objectives

- Define key terms used in the chapter.
- Summarize basic principles of growth and development.
- Discuss the theories of Freud, Erikson, Havighurst, Piaget, Kohlberg, Gilligan, and Fowler.
- Describe the importance of incorporating multiple theories of growth and development in assessing and planning nursing care for individuals and families.
- Describe the dynamics of family in providing nursing care.
- List implications for nursing practice that uses a knowledge base of growth and development.

Key Terms

Accommodation	Faith
Assimilation	Growth and development
Cognitive development	Moral development
Developmental task	Psychosocial theory

Key Topics

The nature of human growth and development.

Principles of human growth and development.

Overview of developmental theories: psychoanalytic theory (Freud), psychosocial theory (Erikson), Developmental tasks (Havighurst), cognitive development (Piaget), moral development (Kohlberg, Gilligan), faith development (Fowler).

Applying growth and development principles and theories to nursing: family dynamics, implications for nurses.

Recurring Displays

Research in Nursing: Growth and Development

Other Significant Displays and Tables

Erikson's Stages of Psychosocial Development (Table 10.2)
Developmental Tasks Described by Robert J. Havighurst (Table 10.3)

Teaching-Learning Activities

Group Activities

1. Ask students, in teams of two to four, to observe various ages at a local shopping mall and report back to the class. Include observations of physical development, dress, and interactions with others.

2. As a group, visit a child-care center and an adult-care center. Spend time interacting with individuals and apply the principles of growth and development. Discuss findings.

3. Using the information from the preceding activity, ask students to identify specific indicators of growth and development from each theorist described in the chapter.

Discussion Questions

1. What did Freud mean by the ego, the superego, and the id?

2. Compare and contrast the developmental theories of Erikson and Havighurst.

3. How do Piaget's theory of cognitive development and Fowler's theory of faith development continue from infancy through adulthood?

4. How do family dynamics affect growth and development?

Writing Activities

1. Ask students to identify and describe examples of ways in which "the rate and pattern of growth and development can be modified".

2. Describe the differences and similarities between the theories of moral development developed by Kohlberg and Gilligan.

Chapter 11
Conception Through Midlife

Learner Objectives

- Define key terms used in the chapter.
- Summarize major physiologic, cognitive, psychosocial, moral, and spiritual development for each age period from conception through the middle adult years.
- List common health problems of each age period from conception through middle adulthood.
- Describe nursing actions to promote wellness at each developmental level.
- Discuss the adult development theories of Gould, Levinson, and Erikson.

Key Terms

Andropause

Anorexia nervosa

Attachment

Bulimia

Child abuse

Denver Developmental Screening Test (DDST)

Failure to thrive (FTT)

Infant

Menopause

Negativism

Neonate

Phase

Play

Prelinguistic

Preschooler

Regression

School-age child

Separation anxiety

Sudden infant death syndrome (SIDS)

Temperament

Toddler

Trimester

Widowhood

Key Topics

Environmental and nutritional influences.

Childhood: conception and prenatal development, the neonate, infancy, toddlerhood, pre-schooler, school-age child (physiologic, cognitive, psychosocial, moral, and spiritual development; common health problems, role of the nurse).

Adolescence: physiologic development, cognitive development, psychosocial development, moral and spiritual development, common health problems, role of the nurse.

Young and middle adulthood: adult developmental theories, young adulthood, middle adulthood (physiologic, psychosocial, cognitive, moral, and spiritual development; common health problems, role of the nurse).

Recurring Displays

Nursing Diagnoses: Childhood, Adolescence, Young to Middle Adult.
Nursing Today: The Child

Other Significant Displays and Tables

Promoting Wellness in Infancy (Table II.2)
Promoting Wellness in Toddlerhood (Table II.4)
Promoting Wellness in Preschoolers (Table II.5)
Promoting Wellness in School-age Children (Table II.6)
Promoting Wellness in Adolescents (Table II.8)
Developmental Tasks of Young and Middle Adults (Table II.9)

Teaching-Learning Activities

Group Activities

1. Ask a panel of nurses representing clinical practice for various age groups to discuss how a knowledge base of normal growth and development is used in safe and holistic client care.

2. Ask students to discuss lifestyles, values, and goals with family members and friends who are in their teens, 20s, 30s, 40s, and 50s; then discuss in a group how each age period is different and similar.

Discussion Questions

1. What health-related risk factors, specific to heredity, environment, and nutrition influence growth and development from conception to midlife?

2. Why are newborn assessments important?

3. What problems in growth and development may appear if bonding does not take place or developmental tasks are not met?

4. What changes have taken place in society regarding an appropriate age for marriage and parenthood?

Writing Activities

1. Ask students to summarize a nursing or psychology journal article that discusses their age group.

2. Ask students to write a descriptive essay about their childhood and adolescence.

3. Ask students to describe their feelings about being an adult, including how these differ from feelings they had about adults as children.

Chapter 12
The Older Adult

Learner Objectives

- Define key terms used in the chapter.
- Describe common myths and stereotypes that perpetuate ageism.
- Gain awareness of own feelings and attitudes toward the aging process and the older adult.
- Compare physiologic and functional changes that occur with normal aging.
- Discuss developmental tasks of the older adult, as described by Erikson and Havighurst.
- Identify socioenvironmental factors in our society that may inhibit the older adult from meeting needs and realizing potentials.
- Discuss nursing implications concerning the continued growth and development of the elderly client.
- List family and community resources that can be utilized to maintain the health and independence of the elderly client.
- Describe the health care needs of the older adult in terms of chronic illnesses, accidental injuries, and acute care needs.

Key Terms

Ageism	Life review
Alternative care	Old-old
Alzheimer's disease	Older adult
Dementia	Reality orientation
Frail-old	Reminiscence
Functional health	Social isolation
Gerontic nursing	Sundowning syndrome
Gerontology	

Key Topics

Aging in our society: Ageism, changing values with a graying population, who is the older adult.

Growth and development throughout the lifespan: physiologic theories, cognitive development, developmental theories (Erikson, Havighurst).

Gerontology and the health care system: meeting health care needs of the older adult, nursing implications.

Recurring Displays

Research in Nursing: The Older Adult
Nursing Diagnoses: The Older Adult
Through the Eyes of a Student
Focus on the Older Adult: Normal Physiologic Changes of Older Adulthood

Other Significant Displays and Tables

Havighurst's Developmental Tasks of Later Maturity
Meeting Needs of the Hospitalized Older Adult

Teaching-Learning Activities

Group Activities

1. Arrange for each student to "adopt" a resident of a local extended care facility and keep a log of observations and communications made during the length of the course.

2. Ask a panel of older adults to discuss changes in their lives as compared to being young and middle adults.

3. Ask a member of the AARP to discuss services provided to older adults.

Discussion Questions

1. Is ageism common? If so, what can be done to decrease the prejudice?

2. Explain why the older adult requires a longer time period to recover from illness or injury.

3. What nursing actions can help maintain orientation and lessen confusion in the hospitalized older adult?

4. What community agencies and support groups are available to help the older adult and family members?

Writing Activities

1. Ask students to describe an elderly family member or person cared for. What physiological changes were present? How and why would the student categorize the individual being described in terms of Erikson's theory?

2. Ask student to outline modifications that can be made in the home of an older adult to promote comfort and safety.

Chapter 13
Loss, Grief, and Death

Learner Objectives

- Define key terms used in the chapter.
- Differentiate the types of loss.
- Describe the grief process and the stages of grief.
- Outline physiologic and psychologic care of the dying client.
- Identify ethical/legal issues concerning death.
- List the clinical signs of approaching death.
- Outline nursing responsibilities following death.
- Discuss the role of the nurse in caring for a client's family.

Key Terms

Actual loss	Loss
Anticipatory loss	Mourning
Bereavement	Perceiving loss
Death	Physical loss
Dysfunctional grief	Psychologic loss
Grief	Terminal illness

Key Topics

Loss and grieving: loss, grieving.

Factors affecting grief and death: developmental considerations, family, socioeconomic factors, cultural influences, religious influences, cause.

Dying: needs of the dying, impact of terminal illness, stages of dying.

Meeting the needs of grieving and dying individuals: clarifying own feelings, assessing needs, communicating.

Promoting self-care and self-esteem: allowing family members to assist in care, meeting client needs, meeting family needs, meeting self needs.

Death: ethical and legal dimensions, clinical signs, nursing responsibilities.

Recurring Displays

Research in Nursing: Loss and Grieving
Nursing Diagnoses: Loss, Grief, and Death
Nursing Guidelines: Facilitating Coping in Grief and Death
Through the Eyes of a Student

Other Significant Displays and Tables

Needs of Grieving Families (Table 13.1)
The Dying Person's Bill of Rights

Teaching-Learning Activities

Group Activities

1. Ask the director of a hospice program to discuss the objectives and services of the program.

2. Ask a nurse specialist responsible for organ donation and transplant teams to present a program on the topic.

3. Ask students to discuss in small groups the feelings they have had from loss. Do they agree with Engel?

Discussion Questions

1. What would you say to the client who says "I'm going to die, aren't I?"

2. Should a terminally ill person be allowed to die at home? Why or why not?

3. How can The Dying Person's Bill of Rights be used when caring for the client who is dying?

4. What are the physiologic manifestations of approaching death?

5. What nursing actions can facilitate family coping with the death of a loved one?

Writing Activities

1. Ask students to describe their feelings and responses to a loss in their life.

2. Ask students to write a brief essay describing the role of the funeral ceremony in coping with loss and grief.

Chapter 14
Introduction to Nursing Process

Learner Objectives

- Define key terms used in the chapter.
- Describe the historical evolution of the nursing process.
- Describe the nursing process and each of its five steps.
- List five characteristics of the nursing process.
- List three client and three nursing benefits of using the nursing process correctly.

Key Terms

Assessing	Nursing process
Diagnosing	Planning
Evaluating	Scientific problem solving
Implementing	Trial-and-error problem solving
Intuitive problem solving	

Key Topics

Historic perspective: evolution of nursing diagnosis.

Description of nursing process: steps of the nursing process, documenting the nursing process.

Problem solving and the nursing process: intuitive problem solving.

Characteristics of the nursing process: systematic, dynamic, interpersonal, goal-oriented, universally applicable.

Benefits of the nursing process

Significant Displays and Tables

Overview of Nursing (Table 14-1)
IIllustration of the Steps of the Nursing Process

Teaching-Learning Activities

Group Activities

1. Ask students, in small groups, to solve an everyday problem (such as finding a book in the library) using (a) trial and error method, (b) the scientific method, and (c) the problem- solving method.

2. Group students in pairs and have them explain the nursing process to each other.

3. Ask a panel of nurses to discuss their use of the nursing process in the clinical setting.

Discussion Questions

1. Summarize each of the five steps of the nursing process.

2. List two personal characteristics you believe will be an asset to your ability to use the nursing process. How can you use your strengths for the remainder of the semester?

3. Why is it important to use the nursing process in caring for clients?

4. Why is the nursing process called a process?

Writing Activities

1. Have students summarize a recent nursing journal article that discusses the nursing process.

2. Ask students to write a paragraph that describes the rationale for the statement: "The nursing process is an interpersonal process."

Chapter 15
Assessing

Learner Objectives

- Define key terms used in the chapter.
- Describe the purposes of the initial nursing assessment and of ongoing nursing assessments.
- Differentiate a nursing assessment from a medical assessment.
- Differentiate objective and subjective data.
- Describe the purposes of nursing observation, interview, and physical assessment.
- Obtain a nursing history using effective interviewing techniques.
- Identify five sources of client data useful to the nurse.
- Differentiate comprehensive admission assessments from focused assessments.
- Plan client assessments by identifying assessment priorities and structuring the data to be collected systematically.
- Identify common problems encountered in data collection noting their possible cause and etiology.
- Explain when data need to be validated and several ways to accomplish this.
- Describe the importance of knowing when to report significant client data and the importance of proper documentation.
- Obtain complete, accurate, relevant, and factual client data.

Key Terms

Assessing	Objective data
Data	Observation
Database	Physical assessment
Interview	Subjective data
Nursing history	Validation

Key Topics

Unique focus of nursing assessment

Data collection: types of data, characteristics of data, data collection methods, sources of data

Planning data collection: comprehensive versus focused data collection, assessment priorities, structuring the assessment

Problems related to data collection

Data validation

Data communication: timing, documentation

Summary points

Recurring Displays

Through the Eyes of a Student

Other Significant Displays and Tables

Common Problems of Data Collection (Table 15-3)
Components of a Nursing History
Nursing Admission Assessment
Gordon's Functional Health Patterns

Teaching-Learning Activities

Group Activities

1. Divide the class into groups of three or four students and have each student interview a client to collect a nursing history using Gordon's functional patterns. Share each member's findings with the group.

2. Perform a visual assessment on the same client and document it using your school's guidelines. Share the results with the group.

3. Group students in pairs and have them take turns interviewing each other about a health related problem they have experienced.

4. Have students use the information from the interview to identify strengths and problems and decide how basic human needs were unmet or partially met.

Discussion Questions

1. What are the differences and similarities between nursing assessment and medical assessment?

2. Define and give examples of objective data and subjective data. What is the difference between these two forms of client information?

3. Describe sources of information (data). Why is the client the best source of information?

4. Why is the validation of information important?

Writing Activities

1. Have students use the interview conducted in Group Activity 3 to write a paragraph describing subjective data and a paragraph describing objective data.

2. Ask students to outline the phases of the nursing interview and briefly describe the nursing responsibilities for each phase.

3. Ask students to write a paragraph describing the critical elements in each phase of the nurse-client interview.

4. Have students list the purposes of the nursing examination.

Chapter 16
Diagnosing

Learner Objectives

- Define key terms used in the chapter.
- Describe the term nursing diagnosis, distinguishing it from a collaborative problem and a medical diagnosis.
- Describe the four steps involved in data interpretation and analysis.
- Use the guidelines for writing nursing diagnoses when developing diagnostic statements.
- List four advantages of using the NANDA approved list of nursing diagnoses.
- Develop a prioritized list of nursing diagnoses using identifiable criteria.
- Describe the benefits and limitations of nursing diagnoses.

Key Terms

Actual problems

Collaborative problem

Cue

Data cluster

Diagnosing

Health problem

Medical diagnosis

Nursing diagnosis

Possible problems

Potential problems

Wellness diagnosis

Key Topics

Unique focus of nursing diagnosis: nursing diagnosis vs. medical diagnosis, nursing diagnosis vs. collaborative problem.

Data interpretation and analysis: recognizing significant data, recognizing patterns or clusters, identifying strengths and problems, reaching conclusions.

Formulating and validating nursing diagnoses: writing diagnoses; what is not a nursing diagnosis; actual, potential (high risk), and possible nursing diagnoses; wellness nursing diagnoses; validating nursing diagnoses.

Documenting a prioritized list of nursing diagnoses.

Nursing diagnosis: a critique.

Significant Displays and Tables

Differentiating Nursing Diagnoses from other Client Problems (Figure 16-2)

Illustration of the Steps of the Diagnostic Process: Data Interpretation and Analysis, Formulation of Tentative Nursing Diagnosis, and Validation of Nursing Diagnosis (Table 16-2)

Examples of Common Errors in Writing Nursing Diagnoses with Recommended Corrections (Table 16-3)

Approved Nursing Diagnoses, North American Nursing Diagnosis Association, 1992

Illustration of the Formulation of Nursing Diagnosis Statement

Teaching-Learning Activities

Group Activities

1. Group the students in pairs. Have one student provide data collected from a nursing assessment done in Chapter 15 and the other student write a prioritized nursing diagnoses list, including both actual and potential high-risk diagnoses.

2. Divide the students in small groups. Ask the students to use a case study to write several possible nursing diagnoses (using the NANDA list) and collaborative problems. Discuss how these diagnoses differ from medical diagnoses.

3. Ask students to use the same case study to cluster groups of data that were used to identify the nursing diagnoses. Would they change any previously-made diagnoses? If so, explain why.

Discussion Questions

1. How do nursing diagnoses differ from medical diagnoses?

2. Explain the statement: "The etiology of the problem directs the nursing interventions."

3. Which section of the PES format is easiest for you to formulate? Which is most difficult?

4. What are the benefits of using the NANDA list in making nursing diagnoses?

Writing Activities

1. Have students summarize a recent nursing journal article that was directed toward a nursing diagnosis.

2. Ask students to describe the difference between an actual health problem and a potential high-risk health problem.

3. Ask students to write a paragraph describing why or why not nursing diagnoses should be made.

4. Ask students to describe how nursing diagnosis relates to assessing.

Chapter 17
Planning

Learner Objectives

- Define key terms used in the chapter.
- Describe the purpose and benefits of planning.
- Identify three elements of comprehensive planning.
- Prioritize client health problems and nursing responses.
- Describe how client goals and nursing orders are derived from nursing diagnoses.
- Develop a plan of nursing care with properly constructed goals and related nursing orders.
- Use criteria to evaluate planning skills.
- Describe five common problems related to planning, their possible causes and remedies.

Key Terms

Client goal (objective/outcome)   Kardex care plan

Computerized nursing care plan   Nursing care plan

Criteria   Nursing order

Discharge planning   Planning

Goal   Standardized care plan

Key Topics

Unique focus of nursing planning.

Comprehensive planning: initial planning, ongoing planning, discharge planning.

Establishing priorities.

Writing goals and developing evaluative strategies: deriving goals from nursing diagnoses, long-term vs. short-term goals, cognitive, psychomotor, and affective goals, guidelines for goal writing, common errors, developing evaluative strategy.

Selecting nursing measures: deriving nursing measures from nursing diagnoses, identifying options, selecting from options, writing nursing orders.

Writing the nursing care plan: formats for care plans, institutional care plans, student care plans.

Care plan controversies.

Problems related to planning.

Summary points.

© 1993 J.B. Lippincott Co., Fundamentals of Nursing:
The Art and Science of Nursing Care

Recurring Displays

Nursing Guidelines: "Guidelines for Writing Goals"
Nursing Guidelines: "Guidelines for Developing the Nursing Care Plan"
Computer Applications in Nursing: "Computer-generated Nursing Care Plans"

Other Significant Displays and Tables

Illustration of Evaluative Statement
Student Care Plan

Teaching-Learning Activities

Group Activities

1. Allow students to work in small groups to read the situation below and respond to the three questions which follow:

   Ann Rogers is a 49-year-old housewife admitted to your unit with low grade fever, multiple joint pains, and complaints of fatigue. She has shortness of breath. She is accompanied by her husband who reports his wife has been feeling poorly for about three weeks.

   1 Prioritize this client's nursing diagnoses.

   2. Write a long-term goal and at least one short-term goal for the priority nursing diagnosis.

   3. Write specific nursing orders for the priority nursing diagnosis.

2. Ask students working in small groups to use a case study to establish both long-term and short-term client goals, and to write nursing orders for priority nursing diagnoses.

3. Give small groups of students a list of standardized nursing orders (for example, "force fluids," "increase activity," "establish trust") and ask them to list as many specific and individualized orders as possible for each standardized order.

Discussion Questions

1. What are five common problems related to planning? Evaluate your plan for any of these problems.

2. What is the purpose of the planning step of the nursing process? Why is it important to include the client and family in the planning step?

3. What are the critical elements of an accurately written client goal?

4. Why is it important to establish priorities of client problems before planning care?

Writing Activities

1. Ask students to define and give examples of the following terms: cognitive goals, psychomotor goals, and affective goals. Identify the place of each goal in the nursing process.

2. Have students use the terms "initial," "ongoing," and "discharge planning" to write a paragraph describing the planning step of the nursing process.

3. Ask students to describe the rationale for making care plan goals client-centered instead of nurse-centered.

Chapter 18
Implementing/Documenting

Learner Objectives

- Define key terms used in the chapter.
- Distinguish independent, interdependent or collaborative, and dependent nursing interventions.
- Use intellectual, interpersonal, and technical skills to implement a plan of nursing care.
- Describe six variables that influence the way a plan of care is implemented.
- Use seven guidelines for implementation.
- Compare and contrast different documentation systems: source- oriented record, problem-oriented record, and computer record.
- Document nursing interventions completely, accurately, concisely, and factually.
- Describe nursing's role in communicating with other health-care professionals by reporting, conferring, and referring.

Key Terms

Change of shift report

Charting by exception

Dependent intervention

Discharge summary

Documentation

Electronic medical record (EMR)

Flow sheet

Graphic sheet

Implementing

Independent intervention

Interdependent (collaborative)

Medication record intervention

Narrative notes

Nursing actions (interventions, measures, strategies)

Nursing care conference

Nursing care rounds

Problem-oriented record (POR)

Progress notes

Protocol

Report

SOAP format

Key Topics

Unique focus of nursing implementation: types of nursing interventions, protocols and standing orders, the nurse as coordinator.

Carrying out the plan of care: prerequisite nursing skills; determining the need for assistance; promoting self care: teaching, counseling and advocacy; assisting clients to meet health goals; a guide for students.

Continuing data collection.

Communicating care: the client record, other communication methods.

Recurring Displays

Nursing Guidelines: "Guidelines for Implementation"

Nursing Guidelines: "Guidelines for Student Clinical Responsibilities"

Nursing Guidelines: "Guidelines for Documentation"

Computer Applications in Nursing: "Computerized Client Care"

Research in Nursing: "Computerized Patient Care Systems - the Benefits of Computerized Documentation via Bedside Terminals"

Through the Eyes of a Student

Other Significant Displays and Tables

Examples of Documentation: Graphic Sheet (Fig. 3)

Activity Flow Sheet with Narrative Notes (Fig. 4)

Problem-Oriented Client Record Forms (Fig. 5)

Charting by Exception Form (Fig. 6)

List of Common Abbreviations and Symbols (Table 18-2)

Teaching-Learning Activities

Group Activities

1. Have students listen to a taped change-of-shift report, and discuss what they learned, what information was most and least helpful, and what they would have done differently.

2. Provide students with a case study that includes independent, interdependent, and dependent nursing interventions. Have students in small groups discuss and categorize the interventions.

3. Using sample client records, have students compare and contrast problem-oriented, source-oriented, and charting by exception client records.

Discussion Questions

1. What are protocols and standing orders? How are they used by nurses?

2. What is the importance of integrating developmental levels into the implementation step of the nursing process?

3. Why are generalizations and subjective observations considered inappropriate in documentation?

4. Discuss the importance of confidentiality concerning client records. How does this confidentiality affect student nurses?

Writing Activities

1. Have students summarize an article from a nursing research journal. How could the findings be used when implementing nursing care?

2. Ask students to write a paragraph explaining the purposes of the client record.

3. Have students list the critical elements in nursing documentation.

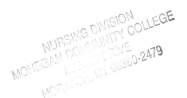

Chapter 19
Evaluating

Learner Objectives

- Define key terms used in the chapter.
- Describe evaluation, its purpose and relationship to other steps in the nursing process.
- Evaluate the client's achievement of goals specified in the plan of care.
- Manipulate factors contributing to the client's success or failure in goal achievement.
- Use the client's responses to the plan of care to modify the plan as needed.
- Explain the relationship between quality assurance programs and excellence in health care.
- Value self-evaluation as a critical element in developing the ability to deliver quality nursing care.

Key Terms

Criteria	process evaluation
Evaluating	outcome evaluation
concurrent evaluation	Nursing audit
retrospective evaluation	Quality assurance program
structure evaluation	Standard

Key Topics

Unique focus of nursing evaluation.

Evaluation criteria and standards.

Measuring client goal achievement: collecting evaluative data, documenting evaluation.

Factors influencing goal achievement.

Modifying the plan of care.

Evaluation program: quality assurance.

Self-evaluation.

Summary points.

Recurring Displays

Computer Applications in Nursing: "Computerized Help in Quality Assurance"
Nursing Today: "Approaches to Quality Health Care: Inspection or Opportunity"
Through the Eyes of a Student

Other Significant Displays and Tables

Common Problems Noted During Evaluation of the Nursing Process (Table 19-1)
Sample Care Plan with Evaluative Statements
Student Checklist for Evaluating Nursing Process Skills

Teaching-Learning Activities

Group Activities

1. Ask students to examine the Kardex on their unit for evaluative statements. In small groups, comment on the findings of your survey of the nursing Kardex.

2. Ask a nurse who is responsible for quality assurance in a health care setting to discuss his or her role and responsibilities.

3. Divide the students into small groups and have students describe a hypothetical client care situation in which evaluation was not done and identify problems that could result in giving care.

Discussion Questions

1. Discuss the importance of the evaluating step in the nursing process.

2. What three options are available to the nurse when evaluating?

3. What is the role of the nursing student in the ANA Quality Assurance Model?

4. Why are time criteria important in the goal statement?

Writing Activities

1. Have students list examples of data that would validate the attainment cognitive, psychomotor, and affective goals.

2. Ask students to summarize a recent nursing journal article that discusses quality assurance or nursing audit.

3. Have students compare and contrast nursing care plans, nursing documentation, and nursing audit.

Chapter 20
Communicator

Learner Objectives

- Define key terms used in the chapter.
- Describe the communication process.
- List at least eight ways in which people communicate nonverbally.
- Describe the interrelationship between communication and the nursing process.
- Identify client goals for each phase of the helping relationship.
- Utilize each of the effective communication techniques when interacting with clients.
- Evaluate self in terms of the interpersonal skills needed in nursing.
- Describe how each of the ineffective communication techniques hinders communication.
- Explain how to facilitate nurse-client interactions in special circumstances.
- Establish therapeutic relationships with clients assigned to your care.

Key Terms

Assertiveness	Message
Body language	Nonverbal communication
Channel	Rapport
Communication	Receiver (decoder)
Empathy	Relationship
Feedback	Semantics
Helping relationship	Source (encoder)
Interpersonal skills	Therapeutic touch
Interviewing techniques	Verbal communication
Language	

Key Topics

The Communication Process: Basic Characteristics of Communication, Forms of Communication.

Communication as a Component of Therapy: Communication and the Nursing Process, The Helping Relationship.

Developing Skills in Communication: Effective Communication, Interpersonal Skills, Assertiveness Skills, Factors Promoting Effective Communication, Blocks to Communication, Communication in Special Circumstances, Documenting Communication.

Recurring Displays

Nursing Guidelines: "Guidelines for Nurses Communicating in Special Circumstances"

Research in Nursing: "Importance of Effective Communication for Families of Critically Ill Clients" and "Nonprocedural and Therapeutic Touch"

Through the Eyes of a Student

Other Significant Displays and Tables

Comparison of Assertive and Nonassertive Behaviors (Table 20-2A)

Teaching-Learning Activities

Group Activities

1. Ask students, working in pairs, to interview each other and tape the interview on video, if available. Ask the class as a whole to critique the session to identify effective and ineffective communication techniques. Use the same interview to identify verbal and nonverbal communications.

2. Arrange students into groups of three and have them alternate being the nurse, the client, and the observer. The observer records the verbal and non-verbal behaviors for a two-minute interaction. The interaction should focus on the nurse's interview of a client problem.

3. Ask volunteers to role-play an interview for the group, identifying orientation, working, and termination phases.

Discussion Questions

1. Have students describe experiences they have had that demonstrate how verbal and nonverbal communications can have very different meanings.

2. Why is the development of interpersonal skills important for nurses?

3. What are your plans for improving your verbal and nonverbal communication techniques?

4. How do gait, posture, and general appearance provide nonverbal communications?

5. Discuss communication skills necessary in special situations: for example, when clients are visually impaired, hearing impaired, unconscious, or speak a language different from the listener's.

Writing Activities

1. Have students describe the three phases of the helping relationship.

2. Have students reflect on the silences that occur during communications. Ask them to describe how they feel and react.

3. Ask students to write a paragraph discussing the statement: "Active listening is hard work."

4. Ask students to use their most recent nurse-client interactions as examples to identify ineffective techniques they used. How could the interactions have been changed to be effective?

Chapter 21
Teacher/Counselor

Learner Objectives

- Define key terms used in the chapter.
- Describe the teaching-learning process, including domains, developmental concerns, and specific principles.
- Describe what factors should be assessed for the learning process.
- Compose diagnoses for identified learning needs.
- Explain how to create a teaching plan for a client.
- Describe what is involved in implementing a teaching plan.
- Name three methods for the evaluation of learning.
- Explain what should be included in the documentation of the teaching-learning process.
- Discuss the nurse's role as a counselor.
- Summarize how the nursing process is used to assist clients in problem solving.
- Describe how to use the counseling role to motivate a client toward health promotion.

Key Terms

Affective learning	Learning readiness
Cognitive learning	Literacy
Contractual agreement	Negative Reinforcement
Counseling	Noncompliance
Developmental crisis	Positive Reinforcement
Formal teaching	Psychomotor learning
Informal teaching	Situational crisis
Learning	Teaching

Key Topics

Aims of teaching/counseling: promoting wellness, preventing illness, restoring health, facilitating coping.

The nurse as teacher: the teaching-learning process.

Nursing process and teaching/learning: assessing the client's learning needs, diagnosing the client's learning needs, planning for learning, implementing the teaching plan, evaluating teaching/learning, documenting teaching/learning.

The nurse as counselor: short-term counseling, long-term counseling, motivational counseling, related nursing diagnoses.

Recurring Displays

Computer Applications in Nursing: "Computer-assisted Instruction (CAI)"

Other Significant Displays and Tables

Sample Teaching Plan (Table 21-1)

Suggested Teaching Strategies for the Three Learning Domains (Table 21-2)

An Analysis of Nursing Responses in Common Counseling Situations (Table 21-4)

Steps in the Teaching-Learning Process

Assessment Parameters: Factors that Affect Learning

Verbs That Can Be Used When Writing Learning Objectives

Teaching-Learning Activities

Group Activities

1. Group students in pairs. Have one student assume the role of nurse for Mrs. Green (student's partner) in the following situation. Then reverse roles. The situation should take 5-10 minutes for each part.

   Sara Green is an 80-year old woman who slipped in the bathtub and fractured her hip. She will be discharged from the hospital soon and wants to return to her home. Mrs. Green lives alone and says she will manage. She refuses to talk to her daughter about placement in a nursing home.

   Jane Black is Mrs. Green's only daughter. Jane works full time to support her family. Jane's husband is recovering from a heart attack and her two children will be going to college next year.

   Jane realizes Mrs. Green will not be able to take care of herself at home. She wants to abide by her mother's wishes but she has many family responsibilities.

   Both Sara Green and Jane Black need help identifying their options and selecting the best choice.

2. Ask a nurse who regularly does client teaching (for example, with diabetic clients or in a prenatal clinic) to present a topic to the class, identifying the organization and methodology used.

3. Ask students to work in pairs to prepare a teaching project for a topic of their own choice, which is directed toward a specific age group. Have them share their projects with the class.

4. Ask students to work in small groups to identify the special learning and counselling needs of persons with AIDS. Identify related nursing interventions.

Discussion Questions

1. Define teaching and learning. Does teaching automatically mean learning has occurred?

2. How does each of the following factors affect teaching: (a) educational level, (b) past and present experiences, (c) physical and emotional status, (d) sensory status, (e) socioeconomic status, (f) motivation?

3. What factors should be considered in developing a teaching plan?

4. How does the role of nurse as a teacher compare to the role of nurse as a counselor?

5. Compare and contrast formal teaching and informal teaching.

Writing Activities

1. Have students analyze their own learning style and describe teaching/learning methods that are most effective.

2. Have students describe a skill they have learned dividing it into cognitive, psychomotor, and affective domains.

3. Ask students to outline a teaching plan for a 12-year-old boy with diabetes who needs to learn how to give himself insulin.

4. Ask students to write a paper which identifies the counselling needs of clients newly diagnosed as HIV+ and suggests related nursing strategies.

Chapter 22
Leader/Researcher/Advocate

Learner Objectives

- Define key terms used in the chapter.
- Describe the teaching-learning process, including domains, developmental concerns, and specific principles.
- Describe what factors should be assessed for the learning process.
- Compose diagnoses for identified learning needs.
- Explain how to create a teaching plan for a client.
- Describe what is involved in implementing a teaching plan.
- Name three methods for the evaluation of learning.
- Explain what should be included in the documentation of the teaching-learning process.
- Discuss the nurse's role as a counselor.
- Summarize how the nursing process is used to assist clients in problem solving.
- Describe how to use the counseling role to motivate a client toward health promotion.

Key Terms

Advance directive	Authoritative knowledge	Objectivity
Advocacy	Scientific knowledge	Planned change
Assertiveness	Traditional knowledge	Power
Autonomy	Leadership	Preceptorship
Change	Autocratic leadership	Professionalism
Change agent	Democratic leadership	Readiness
Durable power of attorney	Laissez-faire leadership	Variable
Group process	Living will	Dependent variables
Informed consent	Management	Extraneous variables
Knowledge	Mentorship	Independent variables

Key Topics

The nurse as leader: leadership dynamics, group dynamics, effecting change through leadership, leadership skills and the nurse's caregiver role.

The nurse as researcher: professionalism of nursing, roots of knowledge, consumerism, caregiver role.

The nurse as advocate: the patient bill of rights, advocacy skills and the nurse's caregiver role.

Recurring Displays

Computer Applications in Nursing: "Personal Computer Databases for Middle Managers"

Nursing Today: "Gender Gap in Research"

Other Significant Displays and Tables

Nursing Research Resources

Checklist for the Beginning Nurse Who Wishes to Develop Leadership, Research, and Advocacy Skills

Teaching-Learning Activities

Group Activities

1. Divide the class into small groups and give students an assignment, such as describing the qualities of the teacher as a leader. Ask students to identify the group dynamics that occurred.

2. Have the group identify a situation in their class/school where change is needed and describe how a class leader might effectively bring about the needed change.

3. Ask a nurse in a management position (in education or in practice) to discuss style of leadership and effective leadership skills with groups.

4. Ask a nurse researcher to present a study, completed or in progress, and discuss its implications.

Discussion Questions

1. Discuss leadership qualities. Why are those qualities important in nursing? How does one develop leadership skills?

2. Compare and contrast the three styles of leadership.

3. How has consumerism influenced nursing research?

4. What is meant by the term mentor?

5. How is research conducted in the unit in which you are working in the hospital?

Writing Activities

1. Ask the students to describe a situation in which a client needed an advocate. Have the students consider the following questions in their response. In what ways could the nurse have been an advocate? Were there alternative methods? Why is being a client advocate important?

2. Have students consider their own leadership qualities, describing their strengths and weaknesses.

3. Ask students to imagine a clinical situation where they are being blamed for something they did not do. Have them describe their feelings and write four or five statements that assertively support their position.

Chapter 23
Vital Signs

Learner Objectives

- Define key terms used in the chapter.
- Discuss nursing responsibilities in assessing temperature, pulse, respirations, and blood pressure
- Compare normal and abnormal vital sign assessments including causes, effects, and implications of abnormal findings.
- Describe the equipment necessary to assess vital signs.
- Identify sites for assessing temperature, pulse, and blood pressure.

Key Terms

Antipyretic

Apnea

Arrhythmia

Bigeminal pulse

Blood pressure

Bradycardia

Bradypnea

Circadian rhythm

Diastolic pressure

Dyspnea

Eupnea

Expiration

Hyperpyrexia

Hypertension

Hypotension

Inspiration

Korotkoff sounds

Lysis

Orthopnea

Orthostatic hypotension

Pulse

Pulse deficit

Pulse pressure

Pyrexia

Respiration

Sphygmomanometer

Stertorous

Stethoscope

Stridor

Systolic pressure

Tachycardia

Vital signs

Key Topics

Frequency of assessing vital signs.

Body temperature: physiologic factors, normal and abnormal body temperature, assessment methods, assessment sites, care of equipment.

Pulse: physiologic factors, assessment methods.

Respiration: physiologic factors, assessment.

Blood pressure: physiologic factors, normal and abnormal blood pressure, assessment methods, assessment sites, alternate techniques.

Care of equipment

Recurring Displays

Focus on the Older Adult: Normal Variations in Vital Signs With Aging
Through the Eyes of a Student

Other Significant Displays and Tables

Mechanisms of Heat Transfer (Table 23.1)
Common Causes of Pyrexia and Its Resolution (Table 23.3)
Various Pulse Rhythms (Table 23.6)
Average and Hypertensive Blood Pressures According to Age (Table 23.9)
Korotkoff Sounds (Table 23.11)

Procedures

Assessing Body Temperature by Oral Method/Glass Clinical Thermometer
Assessing Body Temperature by Oral Method/Electronic Thermometer
Assessing Body Temperature by Rectal Method/Glass Thermometer
Assessing Body Temperature by Axillary Method/Glass Thermometer
Assessing the Radial Pulse Rate
Assessing the Apical Pulse Rate
Assessing the Respiratory Rate
Assessing Blood Pressure

Teaching-Learning Activities

Group Activities

1. Demonstrate and ask students to practice using different types of thermometers, blood pressure apparatus, and stethoscope.

2. Ask each student to work with a partner to assess and record oral body temperature, radial pulse, apical pulse, respirations, and blood pressure.

3. Ask each student to work with a partner to palpate and determine amplitude of pulses at the carotid, brachial, popliteal, and pedal pulse sites.

4. Ask individuals of various ages to volunteer to attend class and have blood pressure taken by students. Discuss differences in findings.

5. Assign students to take a complete set of vital signs on their assigned clients and record the findings on the client's medical record. Discuss these findings with those recorded on admission to the health care setting.

Discussion Questions

1. Why are the processes of radiation, convection, evaporation, and conduction important in nursing care? Describe some specific applications.

2. If a client has an oral temperature of 104° F (40° C) what related assessments should be made?

3. Mr. Jones is unconscious. What route would you choose to take his temperature? What is your rationale for that choice?

4. What factors contribute to tachycardia?

5. What is the physiologic basis for the terms <u>systolic</u> and <u>diastolic</u> when referring to blood pressure?

6. What factors influence blood pressure in a healthy adult?

7. If you take your neighbor's blood pressure three times and each time it is 150/92, what will you do next?

Writing Activities

1. Ask students to write a paragraph describing dyspnea, including nonverbal cues and posture.

2. Ask students to describe the vital signs that would be expected in the following situations: (1) a young woman is brought to the emergency room with severe lacerations, (2) an elderly man has just mowed his yard in 95° heat, (3) a teenage girl faints, and (4) a sleeping baby.

Chapter 24
Nursing Assessment

Learner Objectives

- Define key terms used in the chapter.
- Identify the purposes of the nursing assessment.
- Describe the techniques used during a nursing examination.
- Discuss the importance of client preparation for a nursing assessment.
- Identify equipment used in performing a nursing assessment.
- Describe positioning used for each body system examination.
- Conduct a nursing assessment of each body system in a systematic manner, identifying normal and abnormal findings.
- Document significant findings in a concise, descriptive manner.

Key Terms

Accommodation	Inspection	Rhonchi
Adventitious breath sounds	Jaundice	Thrills
Auscultation	Nasal speculum	Tremor
Bronchial sounds	Ophthalmoscope	Tuning fork
Bruits	Otoscope	Turgor
Bronchovesicular sounds	Pallor	Tympany
Crackles	Palpation	Vaginal speculum
Cyanosis	Petechial	Vesicular breathing sounds
Ecchymosis	Pleural friction rub	Wheeze
Edema	Precordium	
Flushing	Rales	

Key Topics

Health history.

Physical assessment: general guidelines (instruments, positioning, draping), preparing the environment, preparing the client, techniques, general survey.

Assessment of body systems: integument, head and neck, thorax and lungs, cardiovascular and peripheral vascular, breasts and axilla, abdomen, male and female genitalia, rectum and anus, musculoskeletal, neurologic.

Documenting the data.

Recurring Displays

Focus on the Older Adult: Alteration in Physical Assessments With Aging

Focused Assessment Guide: The Internal Eye

Other Significant Displays and Tables

Skin Color Assessment (Table 24.3)

Basic Types of Skin Lesions (Table 24.4)

Glascow Coma Scale (Table 24.6)

Cranial Nerves (Table 24.7)

Grading of Reflexes

Teaching-Learning Activities

Group Activities

1. Demonstrate and ask each student to practice the four techniques of physical examination with a partner.

2. Demonstrate and ask each student to practice selected segments of a physical assessment and record findings. Include general survey, skin, head and neck, thorax and lungs, cardiovascular and peripheral vascular, abdomen, and neurologic assessments.

3. Ask students to complete a complete physical assessment on assigned clients and record the findings in the format used in the health care setting.

Discussion Questions

1. How are the findings from nursing assessment used as part of the nursing process?

2. What terminology can be used to describe abnormal skin lesions?

3. What does a reading of 20/40 for both eyes when using the Snellen chart indicate?

4. What sounds are normally heard when percussing the thorax and abdomen?

5. What is the normal range of motion for the neck, shoulder, and knee?

6. How does the order of assessment techniques differ when assessing the abdomen?

Writing Activities

1. Ask students to choose one of the cranial nerves and describe assessment techniques.

2. Ask students to complete a written documentation of a health history for a classmate.

Chapter 25
Safety

Learner Objectives

- Define key terms used in the chapter.
- Identify factors that may be safety hazards in the client's environment.
- Describe ways in which the client's safety can be promoted in the home and health care setting.
- Identify clients at risk of falling.
- Describe preventive strategies to decrease the incidence of client falls.
- Identify alternatives to using restraints.
- Identify nursing diagnoses associated with a client in an unsafe situation.
- Describe nursing responsibilities for fire safety.
- Identify teaching strategies that should be included in a safety program to prevent poisoning and suffocation.

Key Terms

ground	microshock
incident report	restraint
macroshock	suffocation

Key Topics

Factors affecting safety: developmental considerations, life-style, mobility, sensory perception, knowledge, ability to communicate, health state, psychosocial state.

Assessing safety: the client, the environment, specific risk factors.

Diagnosing.

Planning: client goals.

Implementing: teaching to prevent accidents, considering developmental levels, preventing falls, preventing fires and maintaining fire safety, preventing poisoning, orienting the client to the health agency, preventing equipment-related accidents, preventing procedure-related accidents, filing an incident report.

Evaluating: planning: client goals, implementing, evaluating.

Recurring Displays

Research in Nursing: Making a Difference: Safety

Other Significant Displays and Tables

Developmental Considerations and Safety Topics to be Taught (Table 25-3)
Fire Prevention Checklist for the Home (Figure 25-1)
Checklist for Preventing Falls in the Health Care Facility
Home Modifications to Prevent Risk of Falls
Alternatives to Using Restraints

Procedures

Procedure 25-1   Applying Restraints

Teaching-Learning Activities

Group Activities

1. Demonstrate and have students practice applying and removing restraints (arm, chest).

2. Assess the safety of an assigned client using either Elements of an Environmental Assessment for Falls in the Home or Checklist for Preventing Falls (both in textbook).

3. Ask a representative of a local poison control center to discuss poison prevention measures for different age groups.

Discussion Questions

1. Discuss the risk factors for a safe environment, giving specific examples.

2. Identify high-risk candidates for falls in the health care setting.

3. What teaching can be done in the general public to help prevent fires? Poisoning? Suffocation?

4. What nursing diagnoses are appropriate when meeting safety needs?

5. What are guidelines for nursing actions when caring for a client who is in restraints?

Writing Activities

1. Have students outline a teaching plan for (a) "childproofing" a home against poisoning, or (b) decreasing the possibility of falls for the older adult living at home alone.

2. Have students summarize a nursing or hospital management journal article that discusses environmental safety.

Chapter 26
Asepsis

Learner Objectives

- Define key terms used in the chapter.
- Explain the infection cycle.
- Describe nursing interventions used to break the chain of infection.
- List the stages of an infection.
- Identify clients at risk for developing an infection.
- Identify factors that reduce the incidence of nosocomial infection.
- Identify situations in which hand-washing is indicated.
- Identify nursing diagnoses associated with a client who has an infection or is at risk of developing an infection.
- Differentiate between category-specific and disease-specific isolation systems.
- Differentiate between universal precautions and the body substance isolation system.
- Identify protocols for each isolation system.
- Describe recommended techniques for medical and surgical asepsis.

Key Terms

aerobic
anaerobic
antibacterial
antibody
antigen
antiseptic
asepsis
bacteria
body substance isolation
category-specific isolation system
Centers for Disease Control
convalescent period
disease-specific isolation system

disinfection
endogenous
exogenous
fungi
gram-negative bacteria
gram-positive bacteria
host
iatrogenic infection
immune response
incubation period
infection
inflammatory response
isolation
localized symptoms
medical asepsis

normal flora
nosocomial infection
opportunist
pathogen
prodromal stage
reservoir
resident bacteria or flora
sterilization
surgical asepsis
susceptibility
systemic symptoms
transient bacteria or flora
universal precautions
virulence
virus

Key Topics

Infection: prevention and control: infection cycle, stages of infection, body's defense against infection, factors affecting risk of infection.

Assessing.

Diagnosing.

Planning: client goals

Implementing: using medical asepsis, controlling infectious agents by sterilization and disinfection, using surgical asepsis, using isolation and barrier techniques for infection prevention and control, education about infection control, voicing ethical concerns about infection risks.

Evaluation.

Recurring Displays

Nursing Today: Challenges and Solutions Aids
Through the Eyes of a Student

Other Significant Displays and Tables

Category-Specific Isolation System (Table 26-3)
Basic Practices of Medical Asepsis in Client Care
Basic Principles of Surgical Asepsis
Summary of Universal Precautions: Prevention of Transmission of Human Immunodeficiency Virus, Hepatitis B Virus, and Other Blood-borne Pathogens in Health Care Settings
Body Substance Isolation System

Procedures

Procedure 26-1   Handwashing
Procedure 26-2   Donning and Removing Sterile Gloves
Procedure 26-3   Preparing a Sterile Field
Procedure 26-4   Caring for Client on Isolation Precautions

Teaching/Learning Activities

Group Activities

1. Demonstrate and have students practice the following procedures:

   a. hand washing

   b. putting on sterile gloves

   c. using sterile forceps

   d. opening, maintaining, and adding supplies to a sterile field

2. Have students role-play entering and leaving an isolation unit, wearing cap, mask, gown, and gloves.

3. Role-play the following situation in which three players will be needed: the client, his wife, and the nurse.

   Mr. Sanchez is a newly admitted client who has just arrived from Mexico. He has been placed on enteric isolation precautions. His wife and five children are requesting a visit; he needs to go to X-ray for a chest x-ray. What will you say to his wife? What precautions do you need to take? How will you transport him to X-ray?

Discussion Questions

1. Refer to Group Activity #3. What concerns might you anticipate Mr. Sanchez having regarding his isolation precautions? What would be your response to being assigned to care for Mr. Sanchez?

2. Discuss factors that affect susceptibility to infection.

3. Discuss precautions to prevent transmission of Human Immunodeficiency Virus (HIV).

4. How can health care personnel help reduce the incidence of nosocomial infections?

Writing Activities

1. Have students use their most recent clinical assignment as an example to list the times and reasons for washing one's hands.

2. Have students outline the basic principles of surgical asepsis.

3. Ask students to describe the emotions of clients in isolation and the nursing interventions that are necessary to meet their needs.

Chapter 27
Diagnostic Procedures

Learner Objectives

- Define key terms used in the chapter.
- Describe various diagnostic tests and their purpose.
- Describe nursing responsibilities for a client prior to, during, and following a diagnostic test.
- Discuss the importance of psychological preparation and support to clients having diagnostic tests.
- Identify assessment data appropriate for specific diagnostic tests.
- Evaluate the client's response following a diagnostic examination.

Key Terms

Ascites

Atrioventricular (AV) node

Barium enema

Biopsy

Bronchoscopy

Cholecystogram

Computed tomography

Colonoscopy

Cystoscopy

Depolarize

Electrocardiogram (EKG)

Electroencephalogram (EEG)

Endoscope

Endoscopic retrograde cholangiopancreatography (ERCP)

Fasting state

Esophagogastroduodenoscopy

Fluoroscopy

Intravenous pyelogram

Leads

Liver biopsy

Lumbar puncture

Magnetic resonance imaging (MRI)

Paracentesis

Polarity

Proctosigmoidoscopy

Purkinje system

Radiography

Radioisotope

Radiopaque

Repolarize

Roentgen ray

Sinoatrial (SA) node

Thoracentesis

Transducer

Ultrasonography

Ultrasound waves

Upper gastrointestinal (GI) series

Urinalysis

X-ray

Key Topics

Nursing responsibilities: prior to the test, during the test, after the test.

Diagnostic tests: aspiration procedures, electrical impulse procedures, endoscopic procedures, laboratory procedures, radiography procedures, computed tomography, magnetic resonance imaging, radioisotope scanning, ultrasonography, genetic testing and screening.

Significant Displays and Tables

The Position of the Client and the Site for a Liver Biopsy (Figure 27-3)

The Position of the Client and the Site for a Lumbar Puncture (Figure 27-4)

How Electrical Phenomena Occurring in the Normal Heart appear on the Electrocardiogram (Figure 27-8)

ERCP (Figure 27-11)

Teaching-Learning Activities

Group Activities

1. Have students observe various diagnostic procedures and report back to the class.

2. Ask a radiologist to discuss the preparation, procedures, and significance of findings for radiographic examinations.

3. Role-play the following situation with one student being the client and one student being the nurse.

   Mary Smith is a 40-year-old, married client who is scheduled for the following diagnostic studies: colonoscopy, upper GI series, a barium enema, EKG, and a cholecystogram. Mary asks the nurse:

   a. Can all these tests be scheduled in the same day?"

   b. "What are all these tests for, anyway?"

   c. "Will they hurt?"

   d. "Why does my doctor want to do these tests before he schedules my surgery?"

Discussion Questions

1. Refer to group activity #3. What are the nursing responsibilities for each of the diagnostic tests scheduled for Mary Smith? What other questions would you have if these diagnostic tests were scheduled for you?

2. Discuss general nursing responsibilities before, during, and after diagnostic procedures.

3. Why is psychological preparation an essential nursing intervention prior to diagnostic procedure?

4. Discuss nursing assessments and interventions after a liver biopsy, lumbar puncture, paracentesis, and thoracentesis.

Writing Activities

1. Have students choose one of the diagnostic procedures described in the text and outline a client teaching plan.

2. Have students describe the physiological basis for the P, Q, R, S, and T waves on the electrocardiogram.

3. Ask students to describe the teaching necessary for radiographic studies.

Chapter 28
Continuity of Care

Learner Objectives

- Define key terms used in the chapter.
- Describe the role of the nurse in ensuring continuity of care.
- Discuss considerations for establishing an effective nurse-client relationship when admitting a client to a health-care setting.
- Compare and contrast admission of a client to an ambulatory setting and a hospital setting.
- Discuss transfer of clients within and among health care settings.
- Describe the components of discharge planning in providing continuity of care.

Key Terms

Continuity of care   Discharge planning

Key Topics

The role of the nurse in providing continuity of care.

Admission to a health-care agency: admission to an ambulatory health care facility, admission to the hospital setting.

Transfer within and between setting: transfer within the hospital setting, transfer to a long-term setting.

Discharge planning.

Recurring Displays

Focused Assessment Guide: Discharge Planning Procedures
Admitting a Client to the Unit.
Discharging a Client From a Health Care Agency

Other Significant Displays and Tables

Nursing Admission Data
Discharge Summary

Teaching-Learning Activities

Group Activities

1. Ask a discharge planning nurse to present information on her role and the changing needs of clients as they move from one setting to another.

2. Ask a community or home health nurse to discuss case load, home visits, and reimbursement methods.

3. Ask each student to practice admission procedures and assessments with a partner.

Discussion questions

1. Why is continuity of care so important in meeting the needs of clients requiring health care?

2. What medical procedures are now being done on an out-patient or same-day basis that traditionally were done with clients as in-patients? What implications does this have for nursing?

3. What concerns have you experienced when you entered a health-care setting?

4. What teaching-learning principles must be used when teaching the client and family for self-care at home?

Writing Activities

1. Make a list of nursing diagnoses appropriate for the client who has had abdominal surgery and will be dismissed requiring pain medications, antibiotics, and dressing changes.

2. Write a one-paragraph reaction to a situation in which you are the client and have just been moved from your unit bed to the intensive care unit.

3. Make a list of the information you would want to have if you are the nurse at an extended-care facility and will be admitting an elderly client from the hospital.

Chapter 29
Hygiene

Learner Objectives

- List five functions of the skin, three factors influencing the skin's condition, and four basic principles that guide practices of skin care.
- Identify factors affecting skin condition and personal hygiene.
- Assess the integumentary system and the adequacy of hygiene self-care behaviors using appropriate interview and physical assessment skills.
- Develop nursing diagnoses related to deficient hygiene measures.
- Describe the priorities of scheduled hygienic care, early morning care, morning care, afternoon care, and evening care.
- Demonstrate the back massage, identifying at least four reasons for including the back massage in daily nursing care.
- Demonstrate techniques used when assisting clients with hygiene measures, including those used when administering various types of baths and those used in cleaning each part of the body.
- Describe agents commonly used on the skin and scalp and precautions to observe in their use.
- Plan, implement, and evaluate nursing care for common problems of the skin and mucous membranes.
- Describe the prevention and treatment of pressure ulcers.

Key Terms

Acne	Halitosis	Plaque
Alopecia	Inner canthus	Podiatrist
Caries	Integument	Pressure ulcer (decubitus ulcer, bedsore)
Cerumen	Integumentary system	Pyorrhea
Ceruminal gland	Ischemia	Reactive hyperemia
Dandruff	Necrosis	Sebaceous glands
Dermis	Nits	Sebum
Emollient	Outer Canthus	Shearing force
Epidermis	Pediculicide	Tartar
Erythema	Pediculosis (lice)	
Gingiva	Periodontitis disease	
Gingivitis	Personal hygiene	

Key Topics

Personal hygiene: physiology of the skin, factors affecting skin condition and personal hygiene, nurse as role model, assessing, diagnosing, planning, implementing.

Oral care.

Care of the eyes, ears, and nose.

Hair care.

Nail and foot care.

Perineal and vaginal care.

Nursing process in clinical practice: impaired skin integrity related to pressure ulcer.

Case study.

Recurring Displays

Promoting Wellness: Self-Care: Feminine Hygiene

Focused Assessment Guide

Through the Eyes of a Student

Research in Nursing: Personal Hygiene

Through the Eyes of a Student

Focus on the Older Adult: Risk Factors that Predispose Elderly Clients to a Decubitus Ulcer

Guidelines for Nursing Care: Preventing Pressure Ulcers

Other Significant Displays and Tables

Factors Placing an Individual at High Risk for Skin Alterations (Table 29-2)

Stages of Development of Pressure Ulcers (Figure 29-14)

Procedures

Procedure 29-1   Giving a Bed Bath

Procedure 29-2   Applying Elastic Stockings

Procedure 29-3   Making an Unoccupied Bed

Procedure 29-4   Making an Occupied Bed

Procedure 29-5   Assisting the Client with Oral Care

Procedure 29-6   Providing Oral Care for the Dependent Client

Nursing Process in Clinical Practice

Impaired Skin Integrity: Stage 2 Sacral Pressure Ulcer Related to Incontinence and Malnutrition as Manifested by Persistent Redness and Edema in Sacral Area

Impaired Skin Integrity: Stage 4 Heel Pressure Ulcer Related to Immobility as Manifested by 3-cm Black Necrotic Area on the Left Heel Involving Fascia

Case Study with Nursing Care Plan

Self Care Deficit: Feminine Hygiene, Related to Knowledge Deficit

Teaching-Learning Activities

Group Activities

1. Demonstrate and have students practice the following procedures:
   a. making an unoccupied bed
   b. making an occupied bed
   c. giving a bedbath
   d. providing oral care
   e. applying elastic stockings
2. Ask a diabetic nurse specialist to discuss care of the feet and nails of the diabetic person.
3. Divide students into two groups. Have one group review nursing documentation for the personal hygiene activities that are most routinely performed and one group review nursing documentation for the personal hygiene activities that are least routinely performed. Have each group share their results.

Discussion Questions

1. Have students discuss the following situations:
   a. Agency protocol requires a daily bath, but your assigned client refuses to have one.
   b. Mrs. Jane is a 79-year-old diabetic. During morning care she asks you to soak and trim her toenails.
   c. Mr. Sal has an artificial eye, but is unable to provide self-care.
   d. Miss Mack was in a motorcycle accident a week ago. Her hair is matted together with old blood.
   e. Mr. Toss has an area the size of a quarter on his coccyx that is red and blistered.
2. What is the rationale for the use of anti-embolic stockings? Identify clinical situations in-which they might be used.
3. What are the different types of morning care? How does a nurse decide what type to give?
4. Discuss how skin conditions and personal hygiene are influenced by developmental levels, illness, sociocultural environment, religious beliefs, and personal preferences.

Writing Activities

1. Have students describe their daily personal hygiene habits. How would these change if they were suddenly hospitalized and unable to provide self-care?

2. Have students describe their feelings when they might be assigned to give complete physical care (including perineal care) to a client of the opposite sex. If they have negative feelings, how can they avoid embarrassing both the client and themselves?

3. Have students describe how skin conditions and personal hygiene are influenced by developmental levels, illness, sociocultural environment, religious beliefs, and personal preferences.

Chapter 30
Activity

Learner Objectives

- Define key terms used in this chapter.
- Describe the role of the skeletal, muscular, and nervous systems in the physiology of movement.
- Identify seven variables that influence body alignment and mobility.
- Differentiate isotonic, isometric, and isokinetic exercises.
- Describe the effects of exercise and immobility on major body systems.
- Assess body alignment, mobility, and activity tolerance, utilizing appropriate interview questions and physical assessment skills.
- Develop nursing diagnoses that correctly identify mobility problems amenable to nursing therapy.
- Utilize proper body mechanics when positioning, moving, lifting, and ambulating clients.
- Design exercise programs.
- Plan, implement, and evaluate nursing care related to select nursing diagnoses involving mobility problems.

Key Terms

Abduction	Flaccidity	Passive exercise
Active-assistive exercise	Flexibility	Plantar flexion
Active exercise	Flexion	Pronation
Adduction	Footdrop	Prone position
Aerobic exercise	Fowler's position	Range of motion
Ankylosis	Hemiplegia	Rotation
Atelectasis	Hyperextension	Semi-Fowler's position
Atrophy	Internal rotation	Spasticity
Cartilage	Inversion	Supination
Circumduction	Isokinetic exercise	Supine position
Contractures	Isometric exercise	Sims' position
Dorsiflexion	Isotonic exercise	Synovial joints
Eversion	Ligaments	Tendons
Extension	Osteoporosis	
External rotation	Paraplegia	

Key Topics

Physiology of Movement: skeletal system, muscular system, nervous system, body mechanics.

Factors affecting body alignment and mobility: developmental considerations, physical health, mental health, life-style variables, attitude and values, fatigue/stress, external factors.

Exercise: types of exercise, effects of exercise and immobility on major body systems, role of exercise in preventing illness and promoting wellness, risks related to exercise.

Nurse as a role model.

Assessing: nursing history, physical assessment.

Diagnosing.

Planning: client goals.

Implementing: positioning clients, assisting with range-of-motion exercises, moving and lifting the client, helping clients ambulate, designing exercise programs, teaching exercise benefits to populations at risk.

Evaluating.

Nursing process in clinical practice: activity intolerance, impaired physical mobility, high risk for injury: complications of immobility, alteration in health maintenance: lack of exercise program.

Case study.

Recurring Displays

Research in Nursing: Exercise
Promoting Wellness: Exercise
Focused Assessment Guide: Mobility and Exercise
Nursing Diagnoses for Common Problems: Mobility

Other Significant Displays and Tables

An Overview of the Physical Assessment of Mobility Status (Table 30-4)

Problems of Immobility With Related Etiologies, Assessment Priorities, Client Goals, and Nursing Interventions (Table 30-3)

A Summary and Comparison of the Effects of Exercise and Immobility by Body Systems (Figure 30-8)

Example of a Passive Range-of-Motion Exercise Routine (Figure 30-16)

Procedures

Procedure 30-1	Turning a Client in Bed
Procedure 30-2	Moving a Client Up in Bed (One Nurse)
Procedure 30-3	Transferring a Client from Bed to Stretcher
Procedure 30-4	Transferring a Client From Bed to Stretcher (Three-Carrier Lift)
Procedure 30-5	Assisting a Client to Transfer From Bed to Chair
Procedure 30-6	Transferring a Dependent Client From Bed to Chair (Two Nurses)

Nursing Process in Clinical Practice

Activity Intolerance

Impaired Physical Mobility

High Risk for Injury: Complications of Immobility

Altered Health Maintenance: Lack of Exercise Program

Case Study with Nursing Care Plan

Impaired Physical Mobility (Turning in Bed, Sitting, Standing, Transferring, and Ambulating) Related to Left Hemiplegia and Weakness.

Self-Care Deficit Related to Decreased Alertness and Left-Sided Motor and Sensory Deficits.

Teaching-Learning Activities

Group Activities

1. Demonstrate and have students practice the following procedures:
   a. moving and turning a person in bed
   b. transfers
   c. range-of-motion exercises
   d. ambulating a client
2. Ask a physical therapist to discuss muscle-strengthening exercises and demonstrate crutch-walking.
3. Using Elements of a Mobility/Exercise History and Table 30-3 in the textbook, complete a mobility/exercise assessment on an assigned client.
4. Design, implement, and evaluate an exercise program for participants in a Senior Citizens Center.

Discussion Questions

1. Why is knowledge of the musculoskeletal system and body mechanics important in nursing?

2. Describe proper body mechanics to prevent possible injury to nurses while caring for clients.

3. Compare and contrast isotonic, isometric, and isokinetic exercises.

4. Discuss the positive effects of exercise and the negative effects of immobility on physical and psychosocial needs.

5. An assigned client has a trapeze, trochanter rolls, a footboard, and side rails. Explain the rationale for each of these devices in maintaining alignment.

Writing Activities

1. Have students use each of the following words in a sentence: sprain, dislocation, aerobics, ankylosis, contracture.

2. Have students list ten benefits of regular, moderate exercise.

3. Have students write nursing diagnoses appropriate to problems with activity.

Chapter 31
Rest and Sleep

Learner Objectives

- Define key terms used in this chapter.
- Describe the functions and physiology of sleep.
- Identify 12 variables that influence rest and sleep.
- Describe nursing implications for age-related differences in the sleep-wakefulness cycle.
- Perform a comprehensive sleep assessment using appropriate interview questions, a sleep diary when indicated, and physical assessment skills.
- Describe common sleep disorders noting key assessment criteria.
- Develop nursing diagnoses that correctly identify sleep problems that may be treated by independent nursing intervention.
- Describe nine nursing strategies to promote rest and sleep, and identify their rationale.
- Plan, implement, and evaluate nursing care related to select nursing diagnoses involving sleep problems.

Key Terms

Circadian rhythm

Circadian synchronization

Delta sleep

Electroencephalograph (EEG)

Electromyograph (EMG)

Electrooculograph (EOG)

Enuresis

Hypersomnia

Insomnia

Narcolepsy

Nocturnal myoclonus

Nonrapid eye movement

Parasomnia

Polysomnography

Rapid eye movement (REM)

Rest

Sleep

Sleep apnea

Sleep cycle

Sleep deprivation

Somnambulism

Key Topics

Physiology of sleep.

Factors affecting sleep.

Nurse as role model.

Assessing rest and sleep: sleep history, sleep diary, physical assessment.

Diagnosing.

Planning: client goals.

Implementing.

Nursing Process in Clinical Practice: insomnia, sleep deprivation.

Case Study.

Recurring Displays

Promoting Wellness: Rest and Sleep

Focused Assessment Guide: Rest and Sleep

Nursing Diagnoses for Common Sleep Problems

Research in Nursing: Strategies to Promote Sleep in Elderly Clients

Other Significant Displays and Tables

Characteristics of NREM Sleep (Table 31-1)

Characteristics of REM Sleep (Table 31-2)

Common Sleep Problems: Description and Pertinent Interview Questions (Table 31-4)

Nursing Process in Clinical Practice

Sleep Pattern Disturbance: Insomnia (Difficulty Falling Asleep, Difficulty Remaining Asleep, or Premature Awakening).

Sleep Pattern Disturbance: Sleep Deprivation.

Sleep Pattern Disturbance: Insomnia.

Case Study with Nursing Care Plan

Sleep Pattern Disturbance: Difficulty Falling Asleep and Remaining Asleep Related to New Sleep Environment and Schedule, Evening Caffeine Intake, and Insufficient Meaningful Daytime Activity.

Teaching-Learning Activities

Group Activities

1. Using the questions in the chapter as a guide, ask each student to complete a sleep history with a partner.

2. Have students in small groups discuss their strategies when they are unable to fall asleep.

Discussion Questions

1. Discuss factors in the hospital environment that can interfere with the client's rest and sleep.

2. Compare and contrast REM and NREM, the two major stages of sleep.

3. Define the primary sleep disorders: insomnia, hypersomnia, narcolepsy, and sleep apnea.

4. Discuss variations in sleep patterns across the lifespan.

5. Discuss nursing interventions to promote rest and sleep.

Writing Activities

1. Have students describe their own circadian rhythms. Do they match each student's present lifestyle?

2. Have students briefly describe their own sleep rituals and identify their origin.

3. Have students write nursing diagnoses appropriate for the client with sleep problems.

Chapter 32
Comfort

Learner Objectives

- Define the list of key terms used in the chapter.
- Describe specific elements in the pain experience.
- Compare and contrast acute and chronic pain.
- Identify factors that may affect an individual's pain experience.
- Obtain a complete pain assessment utilizing appropriate interviewing and physical assessment skills.
- Develop nursing diagnoses that correctly identify pain problems and demonstrate the relationship between pain and other areas of human functioning.
- Demonstrate the correct use of non-invasive pain-relief measures: distraction, relaxation, cutaneous stimulation.
- Administer analgesic agents safely to produce the desired level of analgesia without causing undesirable side-effects.
- Collaborate with the members of other health disciplines employing different treatment modalities to promote pain relief.
- Plan, implement, and evaluate nursing care related to select nursing diagnoses for pain problems.
- Utilize teaching and counseling skills to empower clients to direct their own pain management programs.

Key Terms

Acupressure

Acupuncture

Acute pain

Analgesic drug

Chronic pain

Continuous subcutaneous infusion (CSI)

Contralateral stimulation

Cutaneous pain

Cutaneous stimulation

Dynorphins

Endorphins

Enkephalins

Epidural analgesia

Gate control theory

Hypnosis

Imagery

Neuromodulator

Nociceptors

Opioid

Pain

Pain threshold

Pain tolerance

Patient-controlled analgesia (PCA)

Phantom limb pain

Placebo

Psychogenic pain

Referred pain

Relaxation

Somatic pain

Visceral pain

Key Topics

The pain experience: acute versus chronic pain.

Factors affecting the pain experience.

Nurse as role model.

Assessing the pain experience: components of pain assessment.

Diagnosing.

Planning: client goals.

Implementing: establishing a trusting nurse-client relationship, teaching the client about pain, manipulating factors affecting the pain experience, initiating noninvasive relief measures, assisting with pain therapies of other disciplines.

Evaluating.

Nursing process in clinical practice: pain: acute postoperative, chronic.

Case study.

Recurring Displays

Promoting Wellness: Comfort

Focused Assessment Guide: Assessment of the Pain Experience

Nursing Diagnoses for Common Problems: Pain

Focus on the Older Adult: Nursing Strategies for Pain in Older Adults

Research in Nursing: Effective Assessment and Understanding of Pain Promotes Effective Intervention

Other Significant Displays and Tables

Misconceptions and Prejudices About Pain (Table 32-4)

Pain Assessment Tool for Children (Figure 32-4)

PRN Administration of Analgesics (Figure 32-6)

ATC Administration of Analgesics (Figure 32-7)

Clinical Practice Guideline Acute Pain Management: Operative or Medical Procedures and Trauma

Nursing Process in Clinical Practice

Pain: Acute Postoperative

Chronic Pain

Case Study with Nursing Care Plan

Ineffective Individual Coping Related to Irritability, Anxiety, Depression, and Mood Swings

Teaching-Learning Activities

Group Activities

1. Ask nurses from a coronary care unit, an oncology unit, and an acute surgical unit to discuss invasive and noninvasive comfort measures.

2. Have each student work with a partner to practice a relaxation technique.

3. Ask students in small groups to discuss the use of analgesic agents for the following situations:

   a. a newborn infant being circumcised

   b. a known drug addict with a fractured femur

   c. a young adult with terminal cancer

   d. an elderly man with severe rheumatoid arthritis

Discussion Questions

1. What is the gate control theory of pain. Why is it the basis for selected nursing interventions to promote comfort?

2. What is meant by the statement, "Pain is an individual experience?"

3. Discuss physical, environmental, and psychosocial factors that affect the pain experience.

4. What are common misconceptions about pain? How may these misconceptions influence a nurse's plan of care to meet comfort needs?

5. What are some commonly used noninvasive techniques to relieve pain?

6. Discuss the possible rationale for research findings that pain of hospitalized clients is undertreated.

Writing Activities

1. Have students briefly describe personal experiences with pain, including physical and emotional responses.

2. Have students summarize a nursing journal article that discusses nursing interventions to meet comfort needs.

3. Have students write nursing diagnoses appropriate to pain problems.

4. Have students compare and contrast acute pain and chronic pain.

Chapter 33
Nutrition

Learner Objectives

- Define key terms used in the chapter.
- List the six classes of nutrients and explain the significance of each, including variables affecting nutrient requirements.
- Evaluate a diet using the food group approach.
- Identify dietary, medical-socioeconomic, anthropometric, clinical, and biochemical risk factors for poor nutritional status.
- Describe nutritional implications of growth and development throughout the life cycle.
- Perform a nutritional assessment using appropriate interview questions, a 24-hour food recall when indicated, and a nursing examination.
- Describe common nutritional problems noting key assessment criteria.
- Develop nursing diagnoses that correctly identify nutritional problems which may be treated by independent nursing intervention.
- Describe nursing interventions to help clients achieve their nutritional goals.
- Plan, implement, and evaluate nursing care related to selected nursing diagnoses involving nutritional problems.
- Differentiate between the various types of enteral tubes.

Key Terms

Amino acid	Fatty acid	Nitrogen balance
Anorexia	Food and Drug Administration (FDA)	Nutrient
Anorexia nervosa		Nutrition
Anthropometric	Incomplete proteins	Obesity
Basal metabolism	Lipid	Parenteral nutrition
Bulimia	Macromineral	Polysaccharides
Calorie	Macronutrient	Recommended dietary allowance
Cholesterol	Micromineral	
Complete proteins	Micronutrient	Saturated fatty acids
Disaccharides	Minerals	Triglycerides
Enteral nutrition	Monosaccharides	Unsaturated fatty acids

Key Topics

Principles of Nutrition: energy nutrients, regulatory nutrients.

How to choose an adequate diet.

Factors affecting nutrition.

Nurse as role model.

Assessing nutritional status.

Diagnosing.

Planning: client goals.

Implementing.

Evaluating.

Nursing process in clinical practice: altered nutrition: more than body requirement: obesity, altered nutrition; less than body requirement: iron deficiency anemia; knowledge deficit related to a new medical diet.

Case study.

Recurring Displays

Focus on the Older Adult: Nursing Strategies for Nutritional Problems Affecting Older Adults

Promoting Wellness: Nutrition

Focused Assessment Guide: Nutrition

Nursing Diagnoses for Common Problems: Nutrition

Research in Nursing: Nutrition

Other Significant Displays and Tables

Comparison of Nutrition Recommendations for Canada and the United States (Table 33-7)

Cultural Variations on Nutrition (Table 33-9)

The "Food Guide Pyramid" (Figure 33-6)

Elements of a Nutritional Assessment

Nutritional Assessment Considerations for Older Adults

Procedures

Procedure 33-1   Inserting a Nasogastric Tube

Procedure 33-2   Irrigating a Nasogastric Tube

Procedure 33-3   Administering a Tube Feeding

Procedure 33-4   Monitoring a Nasogastric Tube

Procedure 33-5   Removing a Nasogastric Tube

Nursing Process in Clinical Practice

Altered Nutrition: More Than Body Requirements - Obesity

Altered Nutrition: Less Than Body Requirements - Iron Deficiency Anemia

Knowledge Deficit - New Medical Diet

Case Study with Nursing Care Plan9

Altered Nutrition: Less Than Body Requirements, Related to Increased Requirements Imposed by Pregnancy, Nausea and Vomiting, Weight Consciousness, Hurried Schedule, and Food Dislikes.

Teaching-Learning Activities

Group Activities

1. Divide the class into pairs to calculate each other's caloric requirements.

2. Ask a dietitian from a health care agency to discuss special diets and tube feeding formulas.

3. Have each student complete a 24-hour recall and diet history for a partner and identify potential dietary problems.

4. Demonstrate and have students practice inserting and assessing placement of different sizes and types of feeding tubes.

Discussion Questions

1. Discuss the significance, classification, metabolism, source, and functions of carbohydrates, fats, proteins, vitamins, minerals, and water.

2. What physical, psychologic, and socio-economic factors influence nutritional status?

3. Identify nursing diagnoses appropriate to nutritional problems.

4. What assessments would be made to monitor for possible complications for the client who is NPO?

Writing Activities

1. Have students describe their favorite foods and the influence of their family on those choices.

2. Have students write a brief summary of a fad diet they have tried. Why did they stop using that diet?

3. Have students describe what nursing interventions can promote comfort for the client who is NPO.

Chapter 34
Urinary Elimination

Learner Objectives

- Define key terms used in the chapter.
- Describe the physiology of the urinary system.
- Identify seven variables that influence urination.
- Assess urinary elimination, using appropriate interview questions and physical assessment skills.
- Execute the following assessment measures: measure urine output, collect urine specimens, determine the presence of select abnormal urine constituents, determine urine specific gravity, and assist with diagnostic tests and procedures.
- Develop nursing diagnoses that correctly identify urinary problems amenable to nursing therapy.
- Demonstrate how to promote normal urination; facilitate use of the toilet, bedpan, urinal, and commode; perform catheterizations; and assist with urinary diversions.
- Plan, implement, and evaluate nursing care related to select nursing diagnoses involving urinary problems.

Key Terms

Anuria	Incontinence	Residual urine
Catheter	Indwelling urethral catheter	Retention
Condom catheter	Intravenous pyelogram	Retrograde pyelogram
Cystoscopy	Irrigation	Straight catheter
Dysuria	Kegel exercises	Stress incontinence
Enuresis	Micturition	Suppression
Foley catheter	Nocturia	Suprapubic catheter
Frequency	Oliguria	Total incontinence
Functional incontinence	Orthostatic albuminuria	Urge incontinence
Glycosuria	Pneumaturia	Urgency
Hematuria	Polyuria	Urinary incontinence
Hesitancy	Proteinuria	Urination
Hydrometer	Pyuria	Urinometer
Ileal conduit	Reflex incontinence	Voiding

Key Topics

Physiology.

Factors affecting micturition.

Nurse as role model.

Assessing: nursing history, physical assessment

Diagnosing.

Planning: client goals.

Implementing: promoting normal urination, catheterizing theclient's bladder, assisting with urinary diversions

Evaluating.

Nursing process in clinical practice: altered patterns of urinary elimination related to dysuria, altered patterns of urinary elimination related to enuresis, urinary incontinence, urinary retention related to varying etiologies, high risk for nosocomial infection related to indwelling Foley catheter.

Case study.

Recurring Displays

Promoting Wellness: Urine Elimination

Focused Assessment Guide: Urinary Elimination

Nursing Diagnoses for Common Problems: Urinary Elimination

Focus on the Older Adult: Nursing Strategies for Urinary Elimination Problems Affecting Older Adults

Through the Eyes of a Student

Research in Nursing: Urinary Elimination

Other Significant Displays and Tables

Common Diagnostic Procedures Used to Study the Urinary Tract (Table 34-2)

Procedures

Procedure 34-1   Catheterizing the Female Urinary Bladder (Straight and Indwelling)
Procedure 34-2   Catheterizing the Male Urinary Bladder (Straight and Indwelling)
Procedure 34-3   Irrigating the Catheter Using the Closed System
Procedure 34-4   Irrigating the Catheter Using the Open System
Procedure 34-5   Giving Continuous Bladder Irrigation
Procedure 34-6   Applying a Condom Catheter
Procedure 34-7   Changing a Stoma Appliance on an Ileal Conduit

Nursing Process in Clinical Practice

Altered Urinary Elimination Related to Dysuria

Altered Urinary Elimination Related to Maturational Enuresis

Incontinence (Five Types with Varying Causes)

Urinary Retention Related to Varying Causes

High Risk for Infection Related to Indwelling Catheter

Case Study with Nursing Care Plan

Functional Incontinence Related to Difficult Transition to Nursing Home and Mobility Deficit

Impaired Skin Integrity Related to Functional Incontinence

Teaching-Learning Activities

Group Activities

1. Demonstrate and have students practice the following procedures:
    a. use of the bedpan and urinal
    b. insertion of straight and indwelling catheters (male and female)
    c. application of a condom catheter
    d. removing an indwelling catheter
    e. irrigation of an indwelling catheter
    f. measuring specific gravity of urine
2. Ask a laboratory technician to discuss and demonstrate diagnostic examinations of urine.
3. Have students interview and develop an appropriate nursing care plan for an assigned client who has an actual or potential problem with urinary elimination. Share results with class.

Discussion Questions

1. Identify the anatomy and physiology of the urinary system.
2. Discuss developmental, physical, psychosocial, and illness-related factors influencing urinary elimination.
3. Describe guidelines and nursing responsibilities for collecting different types of urine specimens.
4. Identify nursing diagnoses appropriate for problems with urinary elimination.
5. Describe nursing interventions to maintain normal voiding habits for the hospitalized client.
6. What are some samples of nursing interventions to stimulate voiding?

Writing Activities

1. Have students use each of the following words in a sentence: diuretic, hematuria, incontinence, cystoscopy.

2. Mrs. Blue has not voided for eight hours following surgery. Have students write a description of the assessments they will make.

3. Have students outline a teaching plan for teaching self-catheterization.

4. Have students Describe nursing interventions to prevent nosocomial infections in clients who have an indwelling catheter.

Chapter 35
Bowel Elimination

Learner Objectives

- Define key terms used in the chapter.
- Describe the physiology of bowel elimination.
- Identify ten variables that influence bowel elimination.
- Assess bowel elimination using appropriate interview questions and physical assessment skills.
- Assist with the following diagnostic measures: stool collection for laboratory analysis and direct and indirect visualization studies of the gastrointestinal tract.
- Develop nursing diagnoses that correctly identify bowel elimination problems amenable to nursing therapy.
- Demonstrate how to (l) promote regular bowel habits (timing, positioning, privacy, nutrition, exercise); (2) use cathartics, laxatives, and antidiarrheals; (3) empty the colon of feces (enemas, rectal suppositories, rectal catheters, digital removal of stool); (4) design and implement bowel training programs; and (5) use comfort measures to ease defecation.
- Plan, implement, and evaluate nursing care related to select nursing diagnoses involving bowel problems.

Key Terms

Bowel movement	Enema	Laxative
Bowel training program	Feces	Occult blood
Cathartic	Flatulence	Ostomy
Chyme	Flatus	Peristalsis
Colon	Hemorrhoids	Stoma
Constipation	Ileostomy	Stool
Diarrhea	Impaction (fecal)	Suppository
Endoscopy	Incontinence (bowel)	Valsalva maneuver

Key Topics

Physiology.

Nurse as role model

Assessing bowel elimination: nursing history, physical examination, assisting with diagnostic studies.

Diagnosing.

Planning: client goals.

Implementing: promoting regular bowel habits, teaching about cathartics, laxatives, and antidiarrheals, decreasing flatulence, emptying the colon of feces, designing and implementing bowel training programs, meeting needs of clients with bowel diversions, providing comfort measures.

Evaluating.

Nursing process in clinical practice: constipation, bowel incontinence, diarrhea.

Case study.

Recurring Displays

Promoting Wellness: Bowel Elimination

Focused Assessment Guide: Bowel Elimination

Nursing Diagnoses for Common Problems: Bowel Elimination

Focus on the Older Adult: Nursing Strategies for Bowel Elimination Problems Affecting the Older Adult

Research in Nursing: Bowel Elimination

Through the Eyes of a Student

Nursing Guidelines: Inserting a Rectal Suppository

Nursing Guidelines: Changing an Ostomy Appliance

Other Significant Displays and Tables

Diagnostic Studies of the Gastrointestinal Tract (Table 35-3)

Classification of Laxatives (Table 35-4)

Digital Removal of Fecal Impaction (Figure 35-6)

Procedures

Procedure 35-1   Offering and Removing a Bedpan or Urinal

Procedure 35-2   Administering a Cleansing Enema

Nursing Process in Clinical Practice

Constipation

Bowel Incontinence

Diarrhea

Case Study with Nursing Care Plan

Diarrhea Related to Unknown Cause (Possibly Viral, Rule Out Malabsorption of Lactose and Other Causes)

Teaching-Learning Activities

Group Activities

1. Demonstrate and have students practice the following procedures:
   a. the administration of different types of enemas
   b. insertion of a rectal suppository
   c. ostomy care (appliance, irrigations)
2. Ask a nurse who is an enterostomal therapist to discuss ostomy care and teaching.
3. Ask a nurse who works in a rehabilitation or extended care facility to discuss bowel training programs.
4. Ask a radiologist to discuss barium studies of the lower GI tract.
5. Have students interview a client who has an actual or potential problem with bowel elimination. Have them each identify an appropriate nursing diagnosis using the PES format, develop a nursing care plan for this client based on the nursing diagnosis they identified, and implement their nursing plan. Compare results with the class.

Discussion Questions

1. How would you evaluate the effectiveness of your nursing care plan in Group Activity #5?
2. Discuss the anatomy and physiology of the large and small intestine, rectum, and anus.
3. Identify developmental, physical, psychologic, and illness-related factors affecting bowel elimination.
4. Describe the procedures for collecting a stool specimen.
5. What are the nursing responsibilities for the care of clients having endoscopic examinations or x-ray studies of the bowel?
6. Discuss nursing interventions and teaching to promote and maintain normal bowel elimination.

Writing Activities

1. Have the students list ways in which they can promote physical and emotional comfort of a client when meeting bowel elimination needs.
2. Have students outline a teaching plan for diet and exercise to promote normal bowel elimination.
3. Have students write nursing diagnoses appropriate to bowel elimination problems.

Chapter 36
Oxygenation

Learner Objectives

- Define key terms used in the chapter.
- Describe the principles of respiratory physiology.
- Describe age-related differences that influence care of the client with respiratory problems.
- Identify six factors that influence respiratory function.
- Perform a comprehensive respiratory assessment using appropriate interview questions and physical assessment skills.
- Develop nursing diagnoses that correctly identify problems that may be treated by independent nursing interventions.
- Describe 11 nursing strategies to promote adequate respiratory functioning, identifying their rationale.
- Plan, implement, and evaluate nursing care related to select nursing diagnoses involving respiratory problems.

Key Terms

Alveoli	Hyperventilation	Pulse oximetry
Arterial blood gas analysis	Hypoventilation	Rales
Atelectasis	Hypoxia	Residual volume
Bronchodilator	Inhalation	Rhonchi
Cupping	Nasal cannula	Spirometer
Crackles	Nonproductive cough	Suppressant
Cytologic study	Percussion	Sympathomimetic agent
Endotracheal tube	Perfusion	Tracheostomy tube
Expectorant	Phlegm	Ventilation
Fremitus	Pleural friction rub	Vibration
Gurgles	Postural drainage	Wheezes
Hemoptysis	Productive cough	

Key Topics

Physiology of respiration: general principles of respiration, developmental variations.

Factors affecting respiration functioning.

Nurse as role model.

Assessing respiratory functioning: nursing history, physical examination, common methods to assess respiratory functioning.

Diagnosing.

Planning: client goals.

Implementing: establishing a trusting nurse-client relationship,

Promoting proper breathing, promoting and controlling coughing, promoting comfort, providing supplemental oxygen, using artificial airways, assisting ventilation, clearing an obstructed airway, administering cardiopulmonary resuscitation.

Evaluating.

Nursing process in clinical practice: impaired gas exchange, ineffective breathing patterns, ineffective airway clearance.

Case study.

Recurring Displays

Promoting Wellness: Oxygenation
Focused Assessment Guide: Oxygen
Nursing Diagnoses for Common Problems: Respiration
Focus on the Older Adult: Oxygen Problems Affecting Older Adults (DE 36-5)
Research in Nursing: Oxygenation

Other Significant Displays and Tables

Common Methods to Assess Respiratory Functioning (Table 36-2)
Medications Used in Respiratory Functioning (Table 36-3)

Procedures

Procedure 36-1   Administering Oxygen by Nasal Cannula
Procedure 36-2   Administering Oxygen by Mask
Procedure 36-3   Administering Oxygen by Tent
Procedure 36-4   Suctioning the Nasopharyngeal and Oropharyngeal Areas
Procedure 36-5   Suctioning the Tracheostomy
Procedure 36-6   Clearing an Obstructed Airway
Procedure 36-7   Administering Cardiopulmonary Resuscitation on an Adult (One Rescuer)
Procedure 36-8   Administering Cardiopulmonary Resuscitation on an Adult (Two Rescuers)

Nursing Process in Clinical Practice

Impaired Gas Exchange

Ineffective Breathing Pattern

Ineffective Airway Clearance

Case Study with Nursing Care Plan

Ineffective Airway Clearance Related to Exposure to Unknown Antigens, Bronchospasm, Overproduction of Thick Mucus

Teaching-Learning Activities

Group Activities

1. Ask a respiratory therapist to demonstrate and discuss techniques, supplies, and procedures to improve oxygenation.

2. Demonstrate and have students practice the following procedures:
   a. use of the Incentive Spirometer
   b. pursed lip breathing
   c. postural drainage
   d. suctioning

3. Have available for student observation and use:
   a. an Ambu bag
   b. an oxygen flowmeter
   c. various types of oxygen delivery systems
   d. tracheostomy tube

Discussion Questions

1. Identify normal anatomy and physiology of the respiratory system.

2. Discuss developmental, pharmacological, and environmental factors affecting respiratory function.

3. Discuss the effects of cigarette smoking (include both active and passive effects). What environmental controls are being legislated?

4. What over-the-counter medications are commonly used to suppress coughs and help expectorate mucus?

5. Describe nursing interventions to promote comfort and oxygenation.

6. What teaching is necessary to promote safety when oxygen is in use?

Writing Activities

1. Have students summarize a nursing journal article that discusses some aspect of oxygenation.

2. Have students evaluate their own environment (home, work, school, social) for air pollution and describe their findings.

3. Have students write nursing diagnoses appropriate for problems with oxygenation.

Chapter 37
Fluid and Electrolytes

Learner Objectives

- Define key terms used in the chapter.
- Describe the functions of body fluids, the two main compartments where fluids are located in the body, and factors that affect variations in fluid compartments.
- Describe the functions, sources and losses, and regulation of main electrolytes of the body.
- Explain the principles of osmosis, diffusion, active transport, and filtration.
- Describe how thirst and the organs of homeostasis function to maintain fluid homeostasis.
- Describe the role of buffer systems, and respiratory and renal mechanisms in achieving acid-base balance.
- Identify the etiologies, defining characteristics, and treatment modalities for common fluid, electrolyte, and acid-base disturbances.
- Perform a fluid, electrolyte, and acid-base balance assessment.
- Describe the role of dietary modification, modification of fluid intake, medication administration, intravenous therapy, blood replacement, and total parenteral nutrition in resolving fluid, electrolyte, and acid-base imbalances.
- Plan, implement, and evaluate nursing care related to select nursing diagnoses involving fluid, electrolyte, and acid-base imbalances.

Key Terms

Acid	Edema	Metabolic alkalosis
Acidosis	Electrolyte	Milliliter
Active Transport	Embolus	Oncotic pressure
Alkali	Extracellular fluid	Osmolality
Alkalosis	Filtration	Osmosis
Anion	Filtration pressure	PH
Base	Fluid volume deficit	Respiratory acidosis
Blood transfusion	Fluid volume excess	Respiratory alkalosis
Buffer	Hydrostatic pressure	Solute
Cation	Interstitial fluid	Solvent
Cellular fluid	Intracellular fluid	Speed shock
Central venous catheter	Intravascular fluid	Third-space fluid shift
Colloid osmotic pressure	Intravenous fluid	Total parenteral nutrition
Dehydration	Ion	
Diffusion	Metabolic acidosis	

Key Topics

Physiology: body fluids, electrolytes, fluid and electrolyte movement, fluid balance, acid-base balance.

Disturbance in fluid, electrolyte: acid-base balance, fluid imbalances, electrolyte imbalances, acid-base imbalances.

Nurse as role model.

Assessing: nursing history, physical examination.

Diagnosing.

Planning: client goals.

Implementing: preventing fluid imbalances, developing a dietary plan, modifying fluid intake, administering medications, administering intravenous therapy, replacing blood and blood products, giving total parenteral nutrition.

Evaluating.

Nursing process in clinical practice: the surgical client, the oncology client.

Case study.

Recurring Displays

Promoting Wellness: Fluid and Electrolyte Balance

Focused Assessment Guide: Fluid and Electrolyte Balance

Nursing Guidelines: Measuring Fluid Intake and Output

Nursing Diagnoses for Common Problems: Fluid and Electrolyte Balance

Focus on the Older Adult: Fluid Balance in Older Adults

Research in Nursing: Fluid and Electrolyte Balance

Other Significant Displays and Tables

Fluid Intake and Output (Figure 37-7)

Fluid Volume Disturbances: Etiologic Factors, Defining Characteristics, and Nursing Interventions (Table 37-3)

Parameters to be Considered in Clinical Assessment for Fluid, Electrolyte, and Acid-Base Balance (Table 37-7)

Complications Associated with Intravenous Infusions (Table 37-9)

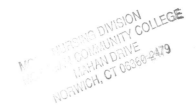

Procedures

Nursing Process in Clinical Practice

Fluid Volume Deficit Related to Fluid Restrictions for Diagnostic Tests or Pathology that Results in Decreased Fluid Intake (Anorexia, Intestinal Obstruction) or Abnormal Fluid Losses (Vomiting, Draining Fistula)

Fluid Volume Deficit Related to Bleeding, Which, if Severe, May Cause Shock and Acute Renal Failure or Actual Fluid Loss and Third-Space Fluid Shift During Surgical Procedure

Fluid Volume Deficit Related to Vomiting, Gastric Suction, or Oral Fluid Restriction Secondary to Ileus Following Abdominal Surgery

Fluid Volume Excess Related to Increased Antidiuretic Hormone Secondary to Surgery and Anesthesia, Aldosterone Secretion, or Overadministration of Isotonic Electrolyte Solutions

Case Study with Nursing Care Plan

Fluid Volume Deficit Related to Prolonged Diarrhea and Decreased Fluid Intake

Teaching-Learning Activities

Group Activities

1. Ask the director of a blood bank to discuss blood donations, type and cross match procedures, and safety measures in blood administration.

2. Demonstrate and have students practice the following procedures:

   a. setting up IV solutions with tubing

   b. starting an IV with an angiocath and a butterfly needle

   c. practice timing and regulating IV rates

   d. changing tubing and solutions

   e. adding a solution to "piggyback" onto a main line

   f. assessing an IV site, and changing IV site dressing

   g. discontinuing an IV

   h. preparing for blood administration

3. Ask an intensive care nurse to discuss arterial blood gases.

4. Have students assess an assigned client's fluid, electrolyte, and acid-base balance using both nursing observations and interview questions from Elements of a Fluid, Electrolyte, and Acid-Base History. Share each student's results with the class.

Discussion Questions

1. Refer to group activity #4. Did you identify any nursing diagnoses for the client you assessed? Support your diagnoses with assessment data.

2. Discuss the functions, compartments, and balance of water in the human body.

3. What assessments are significant in imbalances of sodium, potassium, calcium, magnesium, chloride, bicarbonate, and phosphate?

4. Discuss the buffer systems of the body that maintain normal acid-base balance.

5. Discuss common assessments and interventions for overhydration and dehydration.

6. Describe nursing interventions to maintain or restore fluid and electrolyte balances, including teaching, nutrition, fluid intake and output, administering medications, and/or administering IV therapy.

7. Describe potential transfusion reactions and nursing interventions appropriate to each.

Writing Activities

1. Have students describe how they would reply when Mr. Map says, "I refuse to have the blood transfusion. I'm not going to have AIDS!"

2. Summarize a nursing journal article that discusses fluid, electrolyte, and/or acid-base balance.

3. Have students compare and contrast acidosis and alkalosis.

4. Have students write nursing diagnoses appropriate for fluid, electrolyte, and acid-base imbalances.

Chapter 38
Self-Concept

Learning Objectives

- Define key terms used in the chapter.
- Identify three dimensions of self-concept: self-knowledge, self-expectation, self-evaluation (self-esteem).
- Describe major steps in the development of self-concept.
- Differentiate positive and negative self-concept and high and low self-esteem.
- Identify six variables that influence self-concept.
- Use appropriate interview questions and observations to assess a client's self-concept.
- Develop nursing diagnoses to correctly identify disturbances in self-concept (body image, self-esteem, role performance, self-identity).
- Describe nursing strategies that are effective in resolving self-concept problems.
- Plan, implement, and evaluate nursing care related to select nursing diagnoses for disturbances in self-concept.

Key Terms

Body image   Self-concept

Ideal self   Self-esteem

Personal identity   Social self

Role performance   Subjective self

Self-actualization

Key Topics

Overview of self-concept: dimensions of self-concept, formation of self-concept, threats to self-concept.

Factors affecting self-concept.

Nurse as role model.

Assessing self-concept: self-identity, body image, self-esteem, role performance.

Diagnosing.

Planning: client goals.

Implementing: helping clients identify and use personal strengths, helping high-risk clients maintain a sense of self, changing a negative self-concept, working with parents and educators to develop self-esteem in children and adolescents.

Evaluating.

Recurring Displays

Nursing Diagnoses for Common Disturbances in Self-Concept (Table 38-2)
Promoting Wellness: Self-Concept
Focus on the Older Adult: "Developing Self-Esteem in the Elderly"
Focused Assessment Guide: "Elements Common to a Focused Self-Concept"

Other Significant Displays and Tables

Developmental Changes Affecting Self-Concept (Table 38-1)
High Risk Factors for Self-Concept Disturbances

Nursing Process in Clinical Practice

Body Image Disturbance
Self-Concept Disturbance

Case Study with Nursing Care Plan

Situational Low Self-Esteem related to Decreased Sense of Significance, Competence, Virtue, and Power

Teaching-Learning Activities

1. Ask students to answer the following questions individually: (a) "Who am I?" (b) "Who or what do I want to be?" (c) "How do others see me?" Have them discuss their responses in small groups.

2. Ask a panel of junior and senior high school counselors to discuss adolescent self-concept and the influence of peer pressure.

3. Ask students to interview a hospitalized client to assess self-concept. Use elements common to a Self-Concept Assessment or Defining Characteristics of Low Self-Concept to assist them. Have them discuss their interviews in small groups.

Discussion Questions

1. What are the steps in the development of self-concept?

2. What strategies would you teach parents about the use of the psychological conditions that foster healthy development of the self in children?

3. Discuss how illness alters self-concept and body image. How can the nurse facilitate coping and self-worth?

4. How can nurses facilitate and maintain their own self-concept?

Writing Activities

1. Have students summarize their own strengths. How can these strengths help one personally and professionally?

2. Have students describe a childhood or adolescent learning experience that made them feel good about themselves and motivated them to continue to want to learn.

3. Have students describe stressors on their own self-concepts in their present situation.

4. Have students write a short paper describing what practicing nurses can do to enhance the self-esteem of their colleagues.

Chapter 39
Sensory Stimulation

Learner Objectives

- Define key terms in this chapter.
- Describe the four conditions that must be met in each sensory experience.
- Explain the role of the reticular activating system in sensory experience.
- Identify etiologies and perceptual, cognitive, and emotional responses to sensory deprivation and sensory overload.
- Perform a comprehensive assessment of sensory functioning utilizing appropriate interview questions and physical assessment skills.
- Develop nursing diagnoses that correctly identify sensory-perceptual alterations that may be treated by independent nursing intervention.
- Describe specific nursing strategies to prevent sensory alterations, to stimulate the senses, and to assist clients with sensory difficulties.
- Develop a plan of nursing care to assist clients meet individualized sensory-perceptual goals.
- Implement individualized nursing strategies that successfully resolve the client's individualized sensory-perceptual alterations.
- Evaluate the plan of nursing care using specified criteria.

Key Terms

Arousal	Reception
Auditory	Reticular activating system
Cultural care	Sensoristasis
Deprivation	Sensory deprivation
Gustatory	Sensory overload
Kinesthesia	Sensory-perceptual alterations
Olfactory	Stimulus
Perception	Tactile
Presbycusis	Visceral
Presbyopia	Visual

Key Topics

The sensory experience: components and conditions, arousal mechanisms, sensory alterations.

Factors affecting sensory stimulation.

Nurse as role model.

Assessing sensory functioning: assessing sensory experience, physical assessment.

Diagnosing.

Planning: client goals.

Implementing: preventing sensory alterations and stimulating the senses, meeting the needs of the visually impaired, meeting the needs of the hearing impaired, communicating with a confused person, communicating with an unconscious person.

Evaluating.

Recurring Displays

Nursing Diagnoses for Common Sensory-Perceptual Alterations (Table 39-2)

Focused Assessment Guide: "Elements in a Sensory Functioning Assessment"

Research in Nursing: Appropriate Level of Stimuli

Other Significant Displays and Tables

Overview of Sensory Deprivation and Sensory Overload (Table 39-1)

Suggestions for Stimulating the Senses (Table 39-3)

Under the heading "Implementing" specific guidelines are offered for meeting the needs of clients who are visually impaired, hearing impaired, confused, or unconscious

Nursing Process in Clinical Practice

Sensory Perceptual Alteration: Sensory Deprivation Related to Inadequate Parenting and **Sensory Perceptual Alteration:** Chronic Sensory Deprivation Related to Effects of Aging

Case Study with Nursing Care Plan

Sensory Perceptual Alteration: Mixed Sensory Deprivation and Overload related to Unfamiliar Hospital Environment

(Different Culture) and Stress of Cesarean Birth and Infant's Prematurity

Teaching-Learning Activities

Group Activities

1. Have students work in pairs. Have one student feed a bowl of cereal to a blindfolded partner. Ask students to discuss their feelings as both client and nurse.

2. Ask a speech therapist to discuss the hearing impaired person.

3. Ask a nurse who works on a neurological unit to discuss interventions specific to sensory deprivation or overload.

4. Have students observe the clinical environment for factors that would increase or reduce sensory stimulation. Discuss their findings in small groups.

Discussion Questions

1. What are some factors that place a client at high risk for sensory deprivation?

2. What are some focused interview questions that can be used to assess sensory function?

3. Identify nursing diagnoses appropriate for disturbances in sensory-perceptual function.

4. Discuss nursing interventions and teaching specific to clients who are visually impaired, hearing impaired, confused, or unconscious.

Writing Activities

1. Have students close their eyes for two minutes and describe the sounds, smells, and sensations they receive during that time.

2. Have students evaluate their own family environment as they were growing up. Was it quiet or noisy? What influence did that have on their tolerance of the present environment when they are studying?

3. Ask students to write a paragraph describing factors in the hospital environment that can result in sensory overload.

Chapter 40
Sexuality

Learner Objectives

- Define key terms used in the chapter.
- Describe male and female reproductive anatomy and physiology.
- Describe the sexual response cycle differentiating male and female responses.
- Identify factors that affect an individual's sexuality.
- Perform a sexual assessment utilizing suggested interview questions and appropriate physical assessment skills.
- Describe types of sexual dysfunctions and assessment priorities for each one.
- Develop nursing diagnoses identifying a problem with sexuality that may be remedied by independent nursing actions.
- Describe five areas in which the nurse can provide the client with education to promote knowledge of sexuality.
- Plan, implement, and evaluate nursing care related to select nursing diagnoses involving problems of sexuality.

Key Terms

Abstinence	Lesbian	Rape
Bisexuality	Masturbation	Retarded ejaculation
Coitus	Menarche	Semen
Dyspareunia	Menopause	Sexual dysfunction
Ejaculation	Menses	Sexual harassment
Erectile failure	Menstruation	Sexual intercourse
Erection	Nocturnal emission	Sexuality
Erogenous zones	Orgasm	Sperm
Foreplay	Orgasmic dysfunction	Spermicides
Gay	Ovulation	Sterilization
Heterosexuality	Premature ejaculation	Transsexual
Homosexuality	Premenstrual (tension) syndrome (PMS)	Vaginismus
Impotence		Virginity

Key Topics

Physiology: female, male.

Sexual response cycle.

Sexual expression.

Factors affecting sexuality.

Nurse as role model.

Sexual harassment.

Assessing: sexual history, physical assessment.

Diagnosing.

Planning: client goals

Implementing: establishing a trusting nurse-client relationship, teaching the client, meeting sexuality needs of the hospitalized client, counseling the client regarding sexuality.

Evaluating.

Recurring Displays

Nursing Diagnoses for Common Problems Affecting Sexuality (Table 40-5)
Promoting Wellness
Focused Assessment Guide:
"Elements of a Sexual History"
Research in Nursing: Gender Gap in Research
Research in Nursing: Making a Difference: Women and HIV Infection
Through the Eyes of a Student

Other Significant Displays and Tables

Illustrates and teaches breast self-examination (BSE) (Figure 40-4)
Illustrates and teaches testicular self-examination (TSE) (Figure 40-5)
Developmental Aspects of Sexuality Throughout the Life Span (Table 40-1)
Sexually Transmitted Diseases, Characteristics and Treatment (Table 40-2)
Sexual Dysfunction and Related Nursing Assessment Priorities (Table 40-4)
Sexual Myths and Facts to Refute Them (Table 40-6)
Specific Measures to Stop Sexual Harassment
Model for Counseling Clients with Sexual
Problems (PLISSIT)

Nursing Process in Clinical Practice

Sexual Dysfunction: Inhibited Sexual Desire

Altered Sexuality Patterns: Change in Sexual Expression

Knowledge Deficit: Contraceptive Methods

Disturbance in Self-Concept: Body Image Related to Surgical Removal of a Breast

Case Study with Nursing Care Plan

Knowledge Deficit: Adolescent Sexuality Concerns Related to Misinformation and Absent Family-Based Sex Education

Teaching-Learning Activities

Group Activities

1. Arrange students into groups of three to participate in the following simulation. Students should role-play the characters: a husband, a wife and a nurse.

   Mr. Ruddy is a 55-year-old Black married male who has been hospitalized for a myocardial infarction. Mr. Ruddy is scheduled for discharge tomorrow. You are with Mr. and Mrs. Ruddy at the present time. What is your response to their questions?

   a. "When will we be able to resume sexual activity?"

   b. "Can I hurt my husband during sexual intercourse?"

   c. "We used to have one cocktail before dinner. Can we still do this?"

   d. "I used to take a pill for my blood pressure and I had difficulty achieving an erection. Will this still happen?"

2. Ask a nurse who works in a family planning or women's health clinic to discuss teaching to meet sexual and contraceptive needs.

3. Demonstrate and have students practice the following procedures on models:

   a. breast self-examination

   b. testicular self-examination

   c assisting with a pelvic examination

Discussion Questions

1. Discuss the normal menstrual cycle.

2. How can sexual needs of the hospitalized client be met?

3. Discuss focused interview questions that can be used in ascertaining sexual history.

4. Discuss sexual orientation. How may the nurse's values and beliefs affect the care of a client whose orientation is different than the nurse's?

5. Describe recommended techniques to promote "safer sex." At what age should this information be taught?

Writing Activities

1. Have students describe the age and method in which they learned about male and female sexuality. Did their sex education (formal and informal) help or hinder acceptance of their own sexuality?

2. Have students outline teaching plans for self-examination of breasts and testicles.

3. Have students write a short paper which describes how nursing sensitivity to the sexual needs of clients contributes to better client outcomes.

Chapter 41
Spirituality

Learner Objectives

- Define key terms used in the chapter.
- Identify three spiritual needs believed to be common to all persons.
- Describe the influences of spirituality on everyday living, health and illness.
- Differentiate life-affirming influences of religious beliefs from life-denying influences.
- Distinguish the spiritual beliefs and practices of the major religions practiced in the United States and Canada.
- Identify five factors that influence spirituality.
- Perform a nursing assessment of spiritual health, utilizing appropriate interview questions and observation skills.
- Develop nursing diagnoses that correctly identify spiritual problems.
- Describe nursing strategies to promote spiritual health and state their rationale.
- Plan, implement, and evaluate nursing care related to select nursing diagnoses involving spiritual problems.

Key Terms

Agnostic	Religion	Spiritual needs
Atheist	Spiritual beliefs	Spirituality
Faith	Spiritual distress	

Key Topics

Spirituality and faith.

Spirituality and everyday living: spirituality, health, illness.

Major religions: religions with a western philosophy, religions with an eastern philosophy, native American religions.

Law, ethics, medicine, and religion.

Factors affecting spirituality: developmental considerations, family, ethnic background, formal religion, life events.

Nurse as role model

Assessing spirituality: nursing history, nursing observation.

Planning: client goals.

Implementing: offering supportive presence, facilitating the client's practice of religion, nurturing spirituality, praying with a client, spiritual counseling, referring a client to a religious counselor, resolving conflicts between spiritual beliefs and treatment.

Evaluating.

Nursing process in clinical practice: spiritual distress.

Case study.

Recurring Displays

Nursing Diagnoses for Common Problems of Spiritual Distress (Table 41-3)

Research in Nursing: The Importance of Spirituality to Client Well-Being

Promoting wellness: Spirituality

Focused Assessment Guide: Elements of Spiritual Assessment

Other Significant Displays and Tables

Highlights the Health Care Beliefs and Practices of Western Religions Other Than Those covered in the Text (Table 41-1)

Highlights the Health Care Beliefs and Practices of Eastern Religions (Table 41-2)

Nursing Process in Clinical Practice

Spiritual Distress Related to Deficits in Meaning and Purpose, Love and Relatedness, or Forgiveness

Case Study with Nursing Care Plan

Spiritual Distress Related to Concerns about Relationship with God

Teaching-Learning Activities

Group Activities

1. Ask a panel of religious leaders to present different religious practices, rituals, and beliefs.

2. Have students divide into small groups and discuss the following situations:
   a. A woman who is terminally ill asks, "How could God let this happen to me?"
   b. A client of a very different faith asks you to pray with him.
   c. A client who is a Jehovah's Witness refuses a needed blood transfusion.

3. Divide the students into small groups. Using the Elements of a Spiritual Assessment as a guideline, complete a spiritual assessment on one client. Discuss the results within each group.

Discussion Questions

1. What are the effects of spiritual beliefs on health and illness?

2. What role does spirituality play in the practice of holistic nursing care?

3. What nursing interventions can help the hospitalized client meet spiritual needs?

4. Discuss developmental, family, and life experiences that can influence spirituality

Writing Exercises

1. Have students choose a religion different from their own and describe beliefs and practices that would require adaptation of a plan of care.

2. Ask students to describe how therapeutic communication skills are used to meet spirituality needs.

3. Have students write nursing diagnoses appropriate for spiritual problems

Chapter 42
Medications

Learner Objectives

- Define key terms used in the chapter.
- Discuss drug legislation in the United States and Canada.
- Describe drug names, types of preparation, and types of drug orders.
- Identify drug classifications and actions.
- Discuss adverse effects of drugs, including allergy, tolerance, cumulative effect, idiosyncratic effect, and interactions.
- Obtain client information necessary to establish a medication history.
- Calculate drug dosages, using the various systems of equivalents.
- Describe principles used to safely prepare and administer medications, orally, parenterally, topically, and by inhalation.
- Develop teaching plans to meet client needs specific to medication administration.

Key Terms

Absorption	Iatrogenic disease	Parenteral
Ampule	Idiosyncratic effect	Pharmacodynamics
Anaphylactic reaction	Inhalation	Pharmacokinetics
Antagonist effect	Injections	Pharmacology
Body surface area	Instillation	Piggyback infusion
Bolus	Intradermal	Prefilled cartridge
Chemical name	Intramuscular	Prescription
Cumulative effect	Intravenous	Receptor
Distribution	Irrigation	Subcutaneous
Drug	Medication	Synergistic effect
Excretion	Medication order	Tandem infusion
Generic name	Metabolism	Topical application
Heparin lock	Official name	Trade name

Key Topics

Drug legislation.

Introduction to pharmacology: drug preparations classifications, mechanism of drug action, factors affecting drug action, adverse drug effects.

Assessing: the medication history.

Diagnosing.

Planning for medication administration: medication orders, medication supply systems, dosage calculations, using safety measures while preparing drugs.

Implementing: administering a medication: administering oral medications, administering parenteral medications, administering topical medications, administering medications by inhalation.

Documenting medication administration.

Teaching clients about medication.

Evaluating the client's response to medications.

Recurring Displays

Focus on the Older Adult: Altered Drug Response in Elderly People

Focused Assessment Guide: Medications

Research in Nursing: Strategies to Prevent Nurses from Making Medication Errors

Through the Eyes of a Student

Nursing Guidelines: Applying Topical Medications

Nursing Guidelines: Instilling Eyedrops

Nursing Guidelines: Instilling Nose Drops

Nursing Guidelines: Vaginal Insertion of Suppository or Cream

Other Significant Displays or Tables

Common Abbreviations Used in Prescribing Medications (Table 42-4)

Common Medications That Should Not Be Crushed. (Table 42-5)

The Z-Track Technique (Figure 42-16)

Nursing Responsibilities for Administering Drugs

Common Errors Made in Medication Administration

Procedures

Teaching-Learning Activities

Group Activities

1. Ask a pharmacist to discuss laws and regulations for the administration of controlled substances.

2. Demonstrate and have students practice the following procedures:

   a. reading and understanding medication orders, including abbreviations, symbols, and dosage conversions

   b. administering oral medications in both solid and liquid forms

   c. selecting sizes for needles and syringes, and assembling equipment using sterile technique

   d. withdrawing solution from an ampule and a vial

   e. preparing and using prefilled cartridges

   f. mixing medications in one syringe

   g. locating correct sites for an intradermal, subcutaneous, and intramuscular injection

   h. administering an intradermal, subcutaneous, and intramuscular injection

   i. administering IV medications by piggyback, by bolus, by controlled-volume sets, and by heparin lock

   j. instilling eye and ear drops and ointments

   k. irrigating the eye and ear

   l. inserting a rectal suppository

   m. documenting medication administration

3. Interview a friend or relative to obtain a medication history using Elements of a Medication History.

4. Have students work in groups to complete the following activity on oral and topical medications:

Mary Scott is a 70-year-old woman admitted to your unit. Her medical diagnoses include congestive heart failure and pneumonia. She is to receive the following medications:

Lasix 20 mg p.o. o.d.

Lanoxin 0.125 mg p.o. daily

Ampicillin 500 mg p.o. q.i.d.

Transderm-Nitro patch 5 mg daily

Milk of Magnesia 30 mg h.s. p.r.n. constipation

a. Discuss the principles followed for the safe preparation of oral and topical medications.

b. Simulate the administration of these medications to Mary Scott.

c. Discuss variables that might influence drug action for Mary Scott.

d. List the subjective and objective data you would use to evaluate Mary Scott's response to the medications she has received.

Discussion Questions

1. Why should nurses be familiar with both generic and trade names of drugs?

2. Describe factors that influence drug absorption and action.

3. Discuss different types of drug side effects. What assessments would indicate their occurrence?

4. When may a nurse question a medication order?

5. Describe methods of calculating drug dosages for adults and for children.

6. What are the three checks and the five rights?

7. What safety measures are essential in preparing medications, identifying clients, and administering medications?

8. Describe the steps in combining two types of insulin in the same syringe.

9. Discuss the use of the Z-Track method.

10. Discuss the nurse's responsibility in medication orders.

Writing Activities

1. Have students describe nursing interventions to relieve client discomfort when receiving parenteral medications by injection.

2. Have students outline a teaching plan for use of a nebulizer for administering a drug by inhalation.

3. Have students list the seven parts of a drug order.

4. Have students calculate the medication dosages in the following situations:

a. Mrs. Jones is to receive Demerol 50 mg IM (on hand is a vial containing 100 mg/ml) and Atropine 0.4 mg IM (on hand is an ampule containing 0.4 mg/ml).

b. Baby Brown is to receive Aquamephyton 1 mg IM. It is supplied in a vial containing 1 mg/1 ml.

c. Miss Ross must receive PPD 1 unit intradermally. It is supplied 1 unit/0.1 ml.

Chapter 43
Care of Wounds

Learner Objectives

- Define key terms used in the chapter.
- Describe the physical and psychologic effects of trauma to the body, with resultant wounds.
- Discuss the processes involved in wound healing.
- Describe wound complications, integrating factors affecting wound healing.
- Summarize emergency wound assessment and care.
- Describe the effects of the application of heat or cold.
- Use the nursing process to knowledgeably derive an individualized plan of care for the client with a wound, including the application of dressings and heat or cold.

Key Terms

Abrasion	Dressing	Purulent
Abscess	Evisceration	Retention sutures
Bandage	Exudate	Sanguineous
Binder	Granulation tissue	Scar
Capillarity	Incision	Serous
Closed wound	Laceration	Skin sutures
Compress	Open wound	Stab wound
Contusion	Pack	Wound
Dehiscence	Puncture	

Key Topics

Functions of the skin.

Body's reaction to trauma: wounds, wound healing, wound drainage, factors affecting wound healing, wound complications, psychologic effects.

Nurse's role in wound care: assessing the wound, emergency wound care, implementing (supplies, bandages and binders, dressing change, documenting, staples and sutures), draining wound, special situations.

Heat and Cold Applications: physiologic responses to heat and cold, assessing, diagnosing, planning, implementing (dry and moist heat, dry and moist cold), evaluating

Recurring Displays

Focus on the Older Adult: Factors Affecting Wound Healing in the Older Adult.
Nursing Process in Clinical Practice

Other Significant Displays and Tables

Types of Wounds (Table 43.1)
Benefits of Heat and Cold (Table 43.4)
Emergency Assessments and Care of Specific Wounds
CDC Guidelines for Preventing Infection and Transmission of HIV in Wound Care
Removal of Staples and Sutures

Procedures

Procedure 43-1   Cleaning a Wound and Applying a Clean Dressing
Procedure 43-2   Collecting a Wound Culture
Procedure 43-3   Irrigating a Sterile Wound and Inserting Packing
Procedure 43-4   Applying an External Heating Device
Procedure 43-5   Applying Warm Sterile Compresses to an Open Wound

Nursing Process in Clinical Practice

Mary Cupp, age 35, removal of malignant ovarian tumor, returns to hospital with infected wound.
Alteration in skin integrity

Teaching-Learning Activities

Group Activities

1. Ask a nurse who works in an emergency room to discuss traumatic injuries and emergency care.

2. Ask a nurse who works in an acute surgical unit to discuss different types of dressings.

3. Demonstrate and ask students to practice the following procedures:

   a. handling equipment to remove staples and sutures.

   b. cleaning a wound and applying a sterile dressing.

   c. irrigating a sterile wound and inserting packing.

   d. collecting a wound culture.

   e. applying binders and bandages, using various turns.

   f. applying selected forms of heat and cold.

4. Ask students to provide wound care for assigned clients, and to document wound assessment and care.

Discussion Questions

1. What are the implications of the general principles of tissue healing when planning and implementing care of wounds?

2. What are the three wound healing processes?

3. How can age, wound condition, and health status negatively affect wound healing?

4. What are possible causes and nursing assessments of wound infection, hemorrhage, dehiscence, and evisceration?

5. Why are the local effects of heat and cold useful in wound care?

6. How can skin integrity be maintained for the client with a draining wound?

Writing Activities

1. Ask students to summarize a nursing journal article that discusses some aspect of wound care.

2. Ask students to describe the psychological effects of wounds and scars.

Chapter 44
Perioperative Nursing

Learner Objectives

- Define key terms used in the chapter.
- Describe the surgical experience, including perioperative phases, categories of surgery, types of anesthesia, and informed consent.
- Conduct a preoperative nursing history and nursing examination to identify client strengths as well as factors increasing surgical and postoperative complication risk.
- Demonstrate preoperative exercises: deep-breathing, coughing, and leg exercises.
- Prepare a client physically and psychologically for surgery.
- Describe the nurse's role in the intraoperative phase.
- Identify assessments specific to the prevention of complications in the immediate postoperative phase.
- Plan and implement interventions for ongoing postoperative care to prevent complications, promote a return to health, and facilitate coping with alterations.
- Use the nursing process to knowledgeably develop an individualized plan of care for the surgical client during each phase of the perioperative period.

Key Terms

Atelectasis

Elective surgery

Emergency surgery

General anesthesia

Hemorrhage

Hypovolemic shock

Informed consent

Intraoperative phase

Paralytic ileus

Perioperative nursing

Perioperative period

Pneumonia

Postoperative phase

Preoperative phase

Pulmonary embolus

Regional anesthesia

Shock

Thrombophlebitis

Key Topics

The surgical experience: perioperative period, classification of surgical procedures, anesthesia, informed consent.

Preoperative nursing care: assessing, life-style, diagnosing, implementing (preparing the client psychologically and physically), evaluating.

Postoperative nursing care: immediate care, ongoing care, preventing complications, promoting a return to health, evaluating.

Recurring Displays

Research in Nursing: Perioperative Nursing Care
Focus on the Older Adult: Physiologic Changes With Aging that Increase Surgical Risk
Nursing Process in Clinical Practice

Other Significant Displays and Tables

Classification of Surgical Procedures (Table 44.1)
Preoperative Physical Assessments (Table 44.3)
Preoperative Check List
Postoperative Progress Record
Ambulatory Surgery Assessment Record

Procedures

Procedure 44-1   Preoperative Client Care
Procedure 44-2   Shaving the Skin of the Preoperative Client (dry shave)
Procedure 44-3   Shaving the Skin of the Preoperative Client (wet shave)
Procedure 44-4   Postoperative Care When Client Returns to Room.

Nursing Process in Clinical Practice

Joe Lopez, age 62, has surgical removal of prostate gland.
Anxiety

Teaching-Learning Activities

Group Activities

1. Ask a panel of nurses working in the holding area, operating room, and PAR to discuss nursing roles and client care.

2. Ask a nurse who works in ambulatory surgery to discuss client care specific to this area.

3. Divide students into small groups and ask them to discuss experiences with surgery, either for themselves or for family members.

4. Demonstrate and ask students to practice turning, coughing, deep-breathing exercises, and leg exercises.

5. Ask students to provide pre- and post-operative care for assigned clients based on an individualized plan of care.

Discussion Questions

1. What are the different classifications of surgical procedures?

2. What are the similarities and differences in nursing care for clients with regional and general anesthesia?

3. What effect does preoperative teaching have in reducing anxiety?

4. Why are assessments of respiratory and cardiovascular status especially important in the immediate postoperative period?

5. How can the nurse facilitate coping with alterations resulting from surgery? (provide examples, such as clients with breast removal, amputation, facial surgery, hysterectomy, colostomy).

6. What nursing diagnoses and interventions were used in providing care to surgical clients?

Writing Activities

1. Ask students to write a plan of care with rationale for teaching pain control to the surgical client.

2. Ask students to summarize an article from a nursing journal that discusses some aspect of nursing care for the client having surgery.

3. Ask students to make a list of assessments with appropriate rationale for the client who has just returned to the unit from PAR.